Working
to Live

Michael Nadeau

Carpenter's Son Publishing

Working to Live: Good Health 24/7 Starts From 9 To 5

© 2013 by Michael Nadeau

Published by Carpenter's Son Publishing, Franklin, Tennessee

Writer/Editor: Tammy Kling

Interior Design: Suzanne Lawing

Copy Editor: Andrew Toy

Printed in the United States of America

978-0-9851085-7-1

The journey to create awareness about healthcare and encourage companies to impact employees to become healthier has been profound.

Yet no one can do anything alone. To all of the people I have worked with, done business with, and to my friends and of course my family, thank you for making me better.

FOREWORD

There have always been complexities, both anticipated and not, that have challenged the skill and persistence of even the most competent and courageous of business leaders. Whether it was Henry Ford in the early 20th Century, or Steve Jobs in the 21st, the logistics of bringing an idea to market were certainly challenging, yet in a way, usually surmountable.

But let's be honest.

Business today is different, very different, than what it was thirty, twenty or even ten years ago. The meteoric rise of emerging markets, global expansion and outsourcing, intervention and legislation from every government on earth affecting imports and exports, constant innovations in technology, and the delicate balance of geo-political environments, all combine to require you to never stop thinking, fixing, learning, producing. The simultaneous convergence of all these events rarely kept me up at night ten years ago, but today they do.

And while companies may be assisted by machines, it's important to remember that the heart, soul and gut-wrenching risks are taken by the people who reside within those walls, day-in, day-out; year-in, year-out.

And guess what?

People stress.

When the company is worried, they worry. When the company struggles, they struggle to go the extra mile to pull through the tough times. They give it everything they have, often to the detriment of their personal health and happiness. If we are honest with ourselves as leaders, we'll confess that we've probably fallen into the trap of worrying exclusively about the P&L of Profit and Loss, and sometimes forgot about the "Other P&L" – People and Love. And American employees, as never before, are more stressed-out, more obese, more disillusioned and less healthy than at any other time in our history. For too long, employees have been viewed as only a cost, and sadly, not enough as an investment. And the result of this devaluation is showing.

Mary Kay Ash, who began her company Mary Kay Inc. in 1963, was adamant that profit and loss keeps you in business, but it's the "Other P&L", People and Love, that is just as important. In the fifty years since Mary Kay began her business with only $5,000 in savings, her company has grown into a cosmetics empire, operating in thirty-five countries around the world, with over $3 billion in annual wholesale sales, and over 2.5 million Independent Beauty Consultants and 5,000 corporate employees around the world. All this because of – and not in spite of – a corporate culture built on the Golden

Rule, and the balanced priorities of God first, family second and then career.

But despite our sincere desire to do right for our employees, we, like many companies, were shocked by our out of control healthcare costs. Although that was certainly alarming, something else was even more so: the decreased health of our corporate employees whether working in our warehouses, manufacturing facilities or corporate headquarters. It's as though we could finally see the problem for what it was: not necessarily a broken health insurance system or a lack in offering the right mix of benefits, but rather a broken approach to employee health and overall concern for their well-being.

But this realization didn't happen overnight, but gradually. What is needed to bring about organizational change isn't just a change of thought – but also, a change of heart. In this book, Michael Nadeau offers a glimpse into one such corporate transformation. Instead of the usual textbook approach to the issues that comprise the healthcare crisis, he invites you into a world filled with people who are similar to those you know, and who are struggling with the realities of compromise, priorities and missed opportunities. The bottom line is obvious: a less energized, healthy and passionate employee group results in a less competitive company, and a company with its best days behind it results in an uncertain future for individual families, communities, and ultimately our nation.

But while the story may be fictional, the underlying theory is solid.

There is a saying that goes, "Be the change you want to see." My executive team and I took that saying to heart as never before. And so, several years ago we had a radical shift in the way we viewed healthcare: from one of only fixing illness, to one of promoting health. To that end we partnered with our healthcare providers in a more engaged and strategic way, not just relying on their expertise to handle the day to day paperwork of employee insurance claims, but also relying on their vast resources and network of wellness information, best practices and education. We shifted more accountability and personal responsibility to our employees, inviting them to get fit and active and have provided incentives for them doing so. In an effort to set everyone up for success, we added more healthy choices in our lunchrooms and vending machines, and instituted a Wellness Committee to guide and innovate new ways to keep employees moving. We have walking clubs, and groups that meet for advanced cardio training; we have Weight Watcher groups and groups that simply don't want to gain, but maintain. It's peer pressure, but in all the right ways: everyone helping each other to be the best they can be.

Mary Kay Ash used to say, "Imagine that every person you meet has an invisible sign around their neck that says; Make me feel important." We may be far from perfect, but we're trying. And I think Mary Kay Ash would approve.

David Holl
President and Chief Executive Officer
Mary Kay Inc.

*Healthy citizens are the greatest asset
any country can have.*

—Winston Churchill

INTRODUCTION

Times have changed.

When I was a kid growing up in Northwood, New Hampshire, I ran around the house and yard like most boys throwing the football, or any kind of ball I could get my hands on. My friends and I rode our bikes all over the neighborhood and sometimes we were gone for hours riding from the break of dawn until the sun went down, all summer long. With miles of country roads surrounded by maple trees, there were so many places to explore and a lot of ways to stay active outdoors. We would build elaborate ramps out of old pieces of metal or plywood to jump our bikes. In our imaginations, we were just like Evil Knievel – except that we didn't wear helmets and we didn't suffer anything worse than a skinned knee. We were boys living a full on, active lifestyle. But today, the lifestyle is a lot different.

It's rare to see young children riding their bikes after school, because after school activities are now centered around technology. After a long day at school, the kids want to play with their friends on Xbox, Nintendo, or shared games on a tablet device like the iPad. Playing in the yard is a close second, but the truth is, overall physical activity in adults and children has radically diminished.

Technology reigns, in our fast food nation. Our mobile phones are our office, lifeline, and connection to the world.

And it's not just the level of physical activity that has changed - it's also the way we eat. We aren't farmers anymore, working in the fields and making healthy meals from homegrown vegetables. There wasn't a McDonald's in my town growing up, but now they're everywhere. Everyone I knew ate dinner at home. How did these families manage to cook healthy meals and sit at the table together even with youth sports, after school activities and working moms? Back then, it was the American way. But somewhere along the way the culture changed.

As I got older, I entered the rush and madness of the working world like everyone else, but I never lost my love for sports and any kind of physical activity. I had played soccer and hockey in school, and I enjoyed both so I continued to stay active. Today, I still workout and I want to teach my kids how to live an active lifestyle so they grow up knowing how important it is to stay moving, eat right, and make healthy choices.

What about you?

When people ask me, How did you start this company? It's an interesting story because in one moment sparked by one elevator ride my life (and hopefully many others) changed forever.

I had relocated from Boston to Dallas in 1998 and worked in the IT Consulting industry where we ran technology projects for the "boom" that was going on. Part of my role was to hire and manage our team that was in the field. We grew like crazy, and we hired hundreds of new employees. It was a fun and exciting time, we had a cool culture and we loved what we were doing. I enjoyed the ride we were on but as that bubble began to burst, I knew it was time to consider looking at a new path or career or industry. I was referred to a PEO, (a professional employer organization) and I thought I understood that industry. I thought I knew "HR" because I knew people. I had worked with them, studied them, sold to them, and hired them. It seemed like a great fit, combining my experience outsourcing projects and working with people. So that's what I did. I went to work selling HR outsourcing services to small to midsize employers.

In my short career to this point, I had always worked at companies that were young and energetic. We all seemed to look the same, we played on the softball team together, and drinks after work were the norm. We all hung out like family. But this new job was the first time I was working in what I guess was the "real world," and the demographic wasn't what I was familiar with. Most of my colleagues were stressed or unhealthy or both, and it seemed that 3 out of 4 of my new co-workers were overweight. We had one employee that literally had an oxygen tank in his office. I wondered, is this for real? I was blown away. I went to workout at lunchtime, and the others thought I was odd because of it. I didn't participate in the never-ending birthday parties in the kitchen.

I found myself out there selling these HR outsourcing services to companies and the only ones that were remotely interested were the ones who were looking for cheaper health insurance. The reality of my lack of knowledge of what "HR" was and or is, was never more evident than now. I thought HR was people, culture, your identity. Turns out, it is also the department that generally handles benefits, including the big elephant in the room - healthcare.

I had never thought about healthcare before. I thought of it as something I used when I got hurt playing hockey to fix a broken bone, or my nose. I remember my uncle got leukemia when I was young, and I recall my aunt providing the bone marrow for his transplant. That was healthcare for me, when people were sick. Turns out, more and more of our healthcare costs were driven by people being unhealthy, and it was preventable. I began to wonder, are we killing ourselves?

Why are people not taking care of themselves? In a naïve way, I thought, just eat better, get active and all your troubles disappear. I was wrong again.

The old view of the world began to collapse around me, and I'd go through my day and look at what was happening at work and in society. Childhood obesity, fast food nation, healthcare costs projected to skyrocket.... and then... the elevator ride.

One day I was walking to the elevator to head to lunch. A typical day for me, if I didn't have a sales call, was to go get in a workout at lunch. But today would be different. Our receptionist, who might be one of the sweetest human beings I have ever met, waved me over to the lobby as I was standing by the elevator bank. I opened the glass door and we exchanged typical pleasantries. But something was on her mind. I could see it in her eyes.

"Michael, you work out a lot, do you think you could help me with some exercises?" She raised her arm up and pointed to the dreadful tricep area. She was clearly frustrated, and at a loss on what to do to get in shape.

I thought about the courage it must've taken for an older woman to approach a young man with that question. The embarrassment, anxiety, and helplessness behind such a question hit me square in the heart.

"Sure," I said, "I'll write down some things you can do."

As I got in the elevator and the doors closed, a sadness came over me. Here was a woman who basically asked someone she had only known for a few months, for help.

When I walked away that day, I was shaken. I was shocked by how little she knew about taking that first simple step towards a better life. This was also an interesting time in the world. Obesity began to take center stage as a national problem. The US was getting more and more overweight and unhealthy year after year. National media and attention began to grow and people were taking notice.

That week I offered her some solutions and told her I'd continue to support and encourage her in the coming year. But it was a pivotal moment that illuminated in my mind a need for employees to have positive mentors in the workplace - the place most people spend the majority of their day.

Later, she told me how much that conversation had meant to her.

That single encounter with a colleague caused me to want to help people change their lives. It occurred to me that most people need motivation and guidance to point them in the direction of how to make the right health choices. It seemed crazy to me that employers weren't stepping into the role of creating accountability, encouraging healthier choices, and even rewarding them. Healthcare and the rising cost of providing health insurance to employees had been a growing issue, yet employers weren't stepping up.

At the same time that I was beginning to think about individual health care among employees, a crisis in the workplace was continuing to unfold. The cost of health care was skyrocketing. Carriers weren't providing "health" insurance, they were offering "sick" insurance, and it was only getting worse over time.

You go to the doctor when you're sick. But what if you participated in simple testing to prevent you from getting sick in the first place? What if you could have an environment that supported you in staying healthy, so that preventable conditions never manifested?

Our nation is in a healthcare crisis. And it's my belief that employers can have a big impact by educating employees in order to change the culture, and turn things around.

Yet health is a personal thing. In fact, in most corporations it's taboo to even discuss it. But what if the corporation promoted healthy living? What if the world model changed and the place you spend the most amount of time during the day promoted life, instead of just work?

Increasing individual employee health and care should be a primary initiative for leaders today. I believe the single greatest impact we can have on the healthcare crisis in the United States is through workplace health management programs. Think about it, most people get their insurance through their employer.

I started Viverae with this in mind and it's my personal mission as the leader. I'm not just selling some random product or service. I'm selling a better quality of life. I know that if I can get corporate leaders to embrace prevention programs for their employees, people will live longer, get help when they need it, and enjoy happier, healthier lives without affliction and illness. Time away from the office will be reduced, and so will insurance claims. Insurance costs, medicine, prescription drug addiction and all the very real issues and afflictions you read about will be minimized. The net effect? Individuals can achieve healthier lifestyles while corporations reduce healthcare costs and increase productivity in the culture, and everyone wins.

The name Viverae means to live.

What does that mean to you? For me, living doesn't

mean just to live and be happy in our personal lives. To live means to enjoy every breath, and every experience, no matter where you are. To love your personal life, AND your work life. I don't dread going to work and I don't want my employees to either. I want the work place to be energetic and happy. Where we are all comfortable, more productive, and as a result, our company is profitable. In order for that to happen you've got to have (or begin to create) a positive and healthy culture.

Today, we help corporations reduce their escalating healthcare costs by incorporating health management programs and creating healthier cultures in their workplace. A healthy and happy workforce is a productive and profitable workforce, and increasing preventive healthcare programs decreases the likelihood of depression, mental and physical illness, and high insurance costs.

This is the combination of a Performance Based Health Management approach combined with supporting wellness programs that can transform a culture. I have seen the amazing results and I know we can increase accountability when we work to motivate people to change on a daily basis. The more we touch someone, the greater the chance they are going to become accountable.

How do we do it?

When I first began the process of how to create healthier work environments and cultures, I looked at the traditional approach companies were taking. Basically after years of plan design changes and shopping coverage, the next evolution was to try and make the "wellness" solutions that were in the market available at the workplace. By making "wellness" options a part of the benefit package, the thought was that more employees would take advantage of them because of convenience. The next evolution was to bring risk assessments into the equation. The theory is, people that are in a high state of awareness make better choices and those that are in a low state of awareness make poor choices. When people make bad lifestyle choices, it shows up in the health plan.

I began to look at the risk assessment questionnaires that companies were giving their employees, and noticed right away that they took forever to complete. They were too long or too complex, and most employees didn't complete them! So from the start, you've got minimal participation because someone created a ten page assessment. And the concept of how to get people to participate really began to take center stage. How do we get people motivated, what is the right incentive?

I knew that we could create a process that was

simple. Simplicity is the answer to everything when you're trying to get people to engage. So with the right technology, we created a process that would encourage employees to participate using the technology at their fingertips. Instead of seeing technology as a demon that takes people away from a healthy lifestyle, I knew I could leverage it to help organizations and their employees live better.

Some people wonder if employers should be in the business of wellness. But any employer who is offering a health care plan already is. Employers make decisions each day about employee health. One example is occupational safety. While laws mandate some programs, many employers take extra steps to eliminate safety hazards. Why? Because the short-term cost of prevention is less than the cost of an accident.

Employee health care is the same thing. It's typically the second largest expense on a company's balance sheet behind salary and wages. Employees face the same challenge. How can they control an expense for something so necessary yet unmanageable?

The government mandates that all drivers on the road carry auto insurance. Makes sense right? No one complains about it or thinks it is unfair. When you apply for auto insurance, how do they calculate what you pay? Auto insurance is based on your driving record, which is a reflection of how you have personally performed while driving. Shouldn't health insurance be the same way? Based on how you perform. If you go to the doctor every year, stay healthy, do the right things, should you pay the same as someone who doesn't?

In America, where diabetes and obesity are at an all time high, I feel privileged to be in a business where I can change lives. Sometimes our process has led to preventive testing that has uncovered some very real health problems. This type of preventive testing can help you dig deeper and get other information that helps you solve the problem, instead of leaving it unattended and letting it snowball into a bigger health issue.

Prevention works

At Viverae we provide an employee or member the essential information and programs to achieve that "perfect driving record." In order to know where you need to go and what you need to do, you need a map. This process begins with identifying each person's risk profile, answering questionnaires, participating in annual testing, and review of claims history in order to build a targeted action plan that is personal, meaningful and relevant to each individual's health risks. This data and these plans are all possible because we have an integrated health management system. Combine all of this with the key components of wellness programs, motivation and accountability. Sure the financial incentives around health management usually drive strong participation, but a changed culture will sustain and reinforce this participation.

When people avoid going to the doctor, disease manifests. Studies show that disease such as colon cancer are more treatable, and even preventable, with an early colonoscopy. Diseases like breast cancer and diabetes, two of the most common ailments in our country, can be treated and healed, if they are diagnosed early.

What's all that mean? Prevention works. It's your life, and being intentional about the way you live it can make the difference between life and death, or a high quality life, and an unhealthy one.

Most people are so busy in their personal and professional lives that they live life on autopilot. And it doesn't matter who you are, or what you do. If you are the leader of an organization, you have got even greater responsibilities and demands on your time than the average person. Even if you have the best intentions, it can be difficult to make healthy choices.

For average Americans, a normal day is filled with a barrage of emails, phone calls, work assignments, lists, meetings, texts, family obligations and other activities.

They wake up, have coffee, rush to work, answering emails, text messages and phone calls on the way, work hunched over a computer, eat a fast unhealthy lunch, work some more, and head home. If they're lucky (or intentional about it) they go to the gym, or get a workout in somewhere in between, but statistics on obesity and disease show that the opposite is true. Incorporating physical fitness into the day is a rare occurrence. Most people are simply too tired or stressed to workout after a long day at the office. Add it all up and it can be hard to find time to focus on personal wellness.

They've convinced themselves there aren't enough hours in the day, or they are not disciplined enough to schedule time to exercise. In addition, most people eat poorly, choosing what's quick instead of what's healthiest. They choose fast food and sodas, just because it's convenient, instant gratification, and the antidote to elevated stress hormones (cortisol) and sugar cravings. Instead of taking the time to prepare homemade meals in advance, or go home and make a healthy meal, it becomes easier to order take out.

But the cost is high.

All this under activity and over eating on a weekly basis, creates a rapidly aging population and a sick nation.

Changing attitudes:
driving wellness in the workplace

When imagining the solution to the health crisis, it makes the most sense to start in a place central to the life of nearly every American – the workplace. Most of the 157 million Americans get their health insurance through their employers. Regardless of what happens with health care reform in the United States, both employers and employees will be bearing the brunt of increasing costs for years to come. Yet, by educating ourselves on the three simple things we can do to increase health and longevity—1) regular check ups, 2) eating right, and 3) exercising—it's possible to create change.

And that's why I wrote this book.

If we want to fix the problem we have got to fix the behavior. The answer is to take charge of our own lives and at the same time, urge corporations to take responsibility for supporting healthy lifestyles, choices and habits for their employees.

But can we steer behavior? Naysayers maintain that personal behavior can't be modified or influenced by the workplace. But that is not true. In an environment where people are encouraged through motivation, incentives, and rewards, positive transformation occurs. The popular show *The Biggest Loser*, proves that. When people are incentivized, held accountable, educated, and then rewarded to lose weight, even severely obese people shed pounds quickly. Motivation works.

Even the most elite athletes need a coach. And so do the rest of us!

Most companies understand that benefits are important, and relevant to the workforce, but not as many are actively encouraging their employees to live a healthier lifestyle. In fact some, and maybe even yours, promote working long hours, eating processed foods, late nights out with very little sleep, and little life balance. If you're in a corporate culture where they're not supporting health and wellness, it shows up in the productivity and mindset in employees.

There is another compelling reason that creating good health 24-7 must start from 9 to 5. Because we spend most of our waking hours each week at work, positive behavior changes must be supported there. If progress isn't supported during the 40-plus hours that people spend in offices, factories, warehouses and other worksites, any behavior change will be hard to sustain.

How healthy is your world?

It might sound like a strange question if you've never thought about it. But if you haven't, now is the time. How healthy is your home and workplace? What is your overall health and wellness?

How healthy is the company you work for? Do they promote a wellness lifestyle, positive choices, a healthy office space, and prevention? Does your employer support work life balance and time away from the desk to workout, move your body, and engage your mind in positive activity?

Personal health is a choice. And it's a choice we make each and every day. Overall health is the result of the compound effect of what you eat, how you think, and where you work. In fact, where you work can be one of the most important decisions you'll make when it comes to longevity because that's the place you spend the most amount of time.

Research shows that even the smallest amount of activity and healthy food choices, can increase your lifespan. If an overweight individual loses just 10 percent of their body weight, they can lower blood pressure and cholesterol and improve their health significantly.

This book is a call to action.

Are you ready to make a commitment to a healthier life that will influence those around you? For leaders, it just might make the difference that leads to a cultural shift in America. If you're the CEO of a company, corporate wellness is a commitment you can and should make to your employees.

Today is the day to challenge your beliefs about your lifestyle, your wellness, and the way you'll live out the next decade. By the end of this book, you're going to have a renewed passion for taking control of the way you live. It's your life. If you don't take charge, who will? Have you ever had an a ha moment, where you saw things from a different place and everything shifts? It's my hope that this book is one of those moments for you. This book is going to challenge you to think differently about how you live, and the choices you make.

Leave all afternoon for exercise and recreation,
which are as necessary as reading.
Health is worth more than learning.

—Thomas Jefferson

ONE

John leaned back in the leather chair. The CEO listened for as long as he could, then drew in a deep breath. Executives from his leadership team gathered around the conference table, along with three outside health benefit insurance consultants, for the annual benefits meeting.

John pivoted back and forth in his chair and stared out the window of the seventh floor fishbowl. The conference room spanned one full side of the building, and was surrounded in glass. It had been designed that way intentionally, to create a feeling of openness in the culture. Employees walking by the executive conference room could see the work going on inside, so that the culture displayed transparency, teamwork, and a blending of hierarchies, versus closed doors. John had always wanted it that way. As he looked out the window to the sidewalk below dotted with families walking and riding bikes, he remembered his reasons for building his company. He had wanted to succeed, sure, but more than that he'd wanted to provide a place where others could thrive. He wanted a company where an employee could start in the factory, and rise through the ranks to a management position. He wanted a place where people could be rewarded for their hard work and success. He wanted to give men and women the ability to take care of their families financially, and be proud of what they'd accomplished in life. It was something his own father never had a chance to do.

John turned back to the faces around the table.

It was that time of year. The auto manufacturing company he'd led for more than fifteen years had grown from twelve hundred to three thousand employees. He worked out of corporate headquarters in Sandusky, Ohio, but often visited his factory workers and the other employees scattered throughout three states. Every July he'd meet with his Human Resources and Finance team, along with the consultants, to review the options for the upcoming year.

As the consultants outlined the details in their presentation, he had a flashback to years prior. Each year it was the same. The forecast was grim. Healthcare costs were rising, and there seemed to be no solution.

"We've tried everything," John said. "From switching insurance carriers to plan design changes in order to avoid passing the cost on to our employees."

The CFO leaned forward. He'd been with the company for five years, and was focused on keeping costs down. "Healthcare is about 17 percent of the budget," the CFO said. "We simply can't ignore it when it's the second highest line item."

"That's out of control," John admitted.

"Five years ago we were paying around $4,000 per employee per year, next year we are projected to be over $7,000" the CFO said.

The company employed three hundred people at headquarters, and had a regional distribution center in Syracuse, and two factories in other cities. The two factories employed thousands of men and women in the Midwest and had a strong product line and distribution relationships. But growth had come at a cost.

The consultant spoke up. John liked that he knew their business inside and out. "We've shifted costs around every year, but nothing changes," the consultant said. "The numbers keep rising."

The CEO was frustrated.

"So what are we going to do to contain our healthcare costs?"

"Performance based health management."

"What's that?"

"Each year your organization, like most, has been addressing the problem," the health consultant said "but it's been cost shifting. That's all it is. We need a real solution. A solution that works. And there are proven solutions out there that lead to tangible results."

"Do I have to resign myself to budget seventeen percent every year on healthcare?" John asked, "Or is there a way to reduce that cost?"

Judy, the director of human resources, leaned forward in her seat. The legal representative flipped through a file. Everyone waited for the answer.

"The only way we can contain healthcare costs is to create healthier people," the consultant said. "We need a healthier workforce."

Judy chuckled. "Well, good luck with that. The workforce is stressed, maxed to the limit. Some people are working two jobs at once. Some have been down-sized, roles eliminated, and rolled into one position. Everyone is working longer hours."

John turned in his chair. As much as he hated to ad-mit it, Judy was right. People had been downsized. The culture was stressed, and coming apart at the seams. He looked out the window again, to the brilliant blue sky, the trees. Life wasn't supposed to be stressed. There was more to it than that. He thought of his own father for a brief second, and saw the suit, the briefcase he had always carried to work each day, and then, his mind flashed to the funeral. His father had left for work, dropped dead of a heart attack, and John never saw him again. He was only eleven when it happened.

"Actually," the consultant replied, "it's fairly simple. Other companies we've worked with have seen results by implementing health management programs suc-cessfully. Ultimately it means getting your staff to pay attention to their health, and address their conditions before they turn into major illnesses. That's how we re-duce costs."

"We've tried this in the past," Judy replied. "It didn't work.

John leaned forward in his chair. "Why didn't it work?"

"We had a health fair and HR led it," Judy said. "We also had a mobile cancer screening bus come on site. We've done all that. And nothing changed. We've done it in the past and it never worked out. Participation was low."

"I remember that," said the girl from legal. "I went for an hour and got a free mammogram."

"And while that's good, it's classic wellness. It's a one off event," the consultant said. "It's not a health management plan. It was a good thing to do but it's only a piece of the puzzle. What we are proposing is a program that drives participation with incentives."

"How?" Judy asked. "And I still don't get the distinction. What's the difference between wellness and what you're proposing?"

"There is a distinction between wellness and health management," the consultant replied. "Wellness is a set of singular events that require intrinsic motivation. It's not tied to any external goals. So most wellness programs aren't measurable."

"Explain what you mean about singular events," Judy asked.

"Well, the health fair you mentioned, would be one. Or some companies sponsor 5ks for employees to participate in, and maybe they bring in Weight Watchers, or have Jenny Craig on site another day. Other things to promote wellness would be to supplement gym memberships. They seem like positive events, but it's a one time thing. It's like going to the gym once a month. Won't have any real lasting impact and it's not measurable. Take a mobile mammogram screening day, for instance. People get screened but there's no follow up or system in place for measuring success. A health management program is different. It rewards people to get actively engaged in their health. They're given incentives for participation. They get preventive care, bloodwork, checkups. It's all tracked and measurable. If you don't participate you pay more for coverage." the consultant said.

John thought about it all. There was a lot to digest. Other companies had spent time and money on traditional wellness programs that couldn't measure a return on investment.

"So what do we do?" he asked, exasperated.

The CFO spoke. "Health care costs in general will continue to rise, every year. That's a given. So we need to address this now before it's too late."

John daydreamed. He thought about the why. Why do they do anything? Why implement a health management program? Ultimately, it came down to one word: families. He thought back to the way his father worked hard, long hours, at the expense of family. Before the age of ten he barely saw his father at all.

On the day he first held his own daughter, at the hospital, John figured he'd never live for anything else. His whole life was there in the waiting room. I want her to have a great life, he remembered thinking.

And he thought then that there was no better moment than this. No moment more significant than the birth of a child, than the creation of a new human that had come from him. On that day John vowed to put his family first and work second, and do everything it took to remain healthy so that he could raise his children to be strong, and successful.

John looked at the faces around the conference table. He'd been daydreaming, and now the consultant was speaking.

"Agreed," the consultant said. "When you introduce a health management program you'll address prevention, first. The focus is on engaging the employees, not just enrolling them, in order to affect the change in behavior, and choices, that prevent illness in the first place. But it only works if we get them enrolled AND engaged."

"Health benefits are not negotiable," Judy added.

"We can't just go around making changes to our program."

John interjected. "Change is exactly what we need. We really aren't providing a benefit if all we are doing is paying for disease management after there's a disease. Sounds like we need to be doing more to educate our people about preventing disease."

"We've never had a dedicated health management strategy," the CFO said. "What our consultants are proposing here is linking someone's behavior to what they pay for health coverage."

"Yes," the consultant said. "That's right."

"That's a measurable program where we deliberately set out to enroll, engage, and accelerate the workforce through a program that encourages preventive care, screenings, regular checkups, and an active lifestyle." said the CFO.

John nodded his head in agreement. "It's true that there have been initiatives and events put in place here over the years but none of them have garnered much participation. We've got to get people enrolled, and then incentivize them to continue to be engaged. Participation will be the key to driving real results."

"And how are we going to do that?" Judy asked.

"Incentives are the key to participation. If we are

going to manage the health of the population we need a dedicated health management strategy. The key is participation," the consultant said. "If you are going to have a successful program people need to have skin in the game."

"What does that mean?" Judy asked. "I mean, I get it. We need participation. But how do you get people to care? How do you get them engaged beyond enrollment?"

The consultant drew a diagram on the white board. When he was finished, he stepped back and talked through it, pointing his marker at the circles.

"It's important to tie what employees pay for insurance, to their behavior. If you can tie someone's behavior to what they pay, that's a health management strategy. If we create the right incentive people will participate. If we get high participation, we can reduce risk. If we reduce risk, we reduce cost. Honestly it's no different than the car insurance companies. You get rewarded based on your driving record. If you haven't had any accidents you pay less. Same with the credit score system. You want a higher credit limit? Your spending behavior has to warrant it. And you've got to pay your bills on time."

"That's an interesting way to look at it," said the

CFO. "especially when it comes to healthcare. Because what you're really talking about is rewarding employees based on compliance."

"Exactly!" the consultant said. "And why shouldn't you shift dollars to the unhealthy people? It's their choice to earn money back on their insurance premium or not. Ultimately you're creating an incentive program to get healthy. It's not about wellness. It's about managing your health and equipping employees to make better decisions."

John sat up in his chair. They had his attention now. Everything they'd said made sense. He began to wonder why he hadn't implemented something sooner.

"We can build a program that requires people to participate," the consultant said.

"Is that discrimination?" the legal assistant asked.

"No," the consultant answered. "because the programs are voluntary. They exist in companies across America. And they're working. As long as the contribution rates are equal for everyone it's fine."

"I read somewhere that 75% of healthcare costs are preventable," the legal department manager said. "Is that true?"

"Yes. It adds up. Last year alone, more than 8 million dollars of what you spent falls under the category of preventable."

The CEO stood and walked to the front of the room.

"It's clear to me that we have to do this. It's our only option, and honestly, it makes sense." He looked at the consultant. "It's time to implement a health management program. Performance based health management gives people the opportunity to pay less, based on their behavior."

TWO

In the days after the meeting John began seeing things in a different way. Before, he hadn't noticed the strained faces in his employees. He hadn't seen how some worked late into the night just to get everything done, while others skipped lunch to squeeze in extra hours. But now as he passed through the hallways he noticed all of these things. His employees walked quickly, as if they were stressed and overworked. An overweight man passed by in the hallway, his eyes glued to his cellphone, texting. He didn't acknowledge John at all. A young girl wearing wrinkled jeans and sneakers walked by quickly and disappeared into a cubicle. Where were the smiles? What had happened to the fun, professional, enthusiastic people he'd hired?

John headed towards the elevator. The meeting with his consultants was a breakthrough and he had thought about it every day since. A performance based health management program would be good for his team, but also for his clients. His employees had to be their best physically and mentally in order to work at peak performance. How could they give their best to the clients, if they didn't feel their best? He felt like a health management program would not only reduce workers' compensation and short term disability claims, but that it would reduce absenteeism. It would impact productivity by encouraging healthier choices.

He'd have a healthier workforce as a result. At the factories, workers' compensation claims had been at an all time high. He wondered if it would've been reduced with the proper focus on safety and preventive measures, with the help of the corporate healthcare program facilitator. He was convinced it was time to make the change.

Implementing a health management program was

the right move, but it was also time to think about all of the little things that the company did early on. Making wellness a priority in the culture was a must. It was time to get the energy in the company back.

Early on, he had noticed a vibrant energy. The employees were young and aggressive, and many ran the stairs or walked the sidewalks surrounding the building during their lunch hour. There was a vibrant, can do spirit all around.

But lately, he hadn't seen any of that. In fact, it had been years. He'd been so wrapped up in working long nights and building the business that he hadn't invested in his culture the way he should have. It became clear that his culture was getting away from him and it was time for the company to take control before it got worse.

John felt a headache pressing against his temple. He hadn't eaten yet, and before the elevator doors could completely open a small crowd filtered out, and he rushed in and bumped into Eleanor from Accounting. Her papers fell to the floor, and everyone rushed to gather them which created more chaos. A girl he'd never seen before wearing a company badge dropped her cellphone and keys. She was a large girl in her thirties.

Standing beside her was Don, one of his top executives. They'd golfed together so much that he considered him a close friend, as well as an employee. They exchanged hellos, and the CEO noticed he smelled like cigarettes. It was strong, and lingered.

"I'm so sorry," Eleanor said to no one in particular. She was nearly sixty, but she blushed like a seventeen year old.

The CEO smiled. "It was my fault," he said.

Eleanor kneeled over for the documents and when she stood back up she was out of breath. She stumbled backwards and he grabbed her elbow, and held her up.

"Are you okay?" he asked.

She waved her hand in front of her, in a gesture that said she needed a minute. It was something his mom used to do.

The CEO held her arm steady and waited patiently, as she leaned against the wall. He thought about what would happen if she had a heart attack right there on the spot. She was probably the oldest employee he had.

Angela from client services passed by on her way to a meeting. She was a 35 year old single mom who had risen through the ranks. She seemed rushed. "Everything okay here?" she asked, concerned.

Eleanor waved it away. "It's nothing," she said. "I just need to catch my breath."

The CEO walked the woman back to her office in slow, agonizing steps and waited while she gathered her things. He arranged for his assistant to drive her home, and suggested she take the rest of the day off.

Later that night he went home, poured himself a glass of scotch and sat in his study to read. He felt anxious, yet he couldn't really pinpoint why. His thoughts jumped restlessly from his finances, to the company, to his twenty three year old daughter who was relocating to New York for her new job. He checked his stocks on the tablet, and then sifted through email. One problem after another. An email from his director of sales, and another from his ex-wife. One from his accountant and another from a client. None of it bad news but none of it good.

He took another sip of the scotch and exhaled. He felt tense. He picked up the newspaper and read an article on the front page of The Wall Street Journal. The writer talked about how happiness in the workforce translated to results. Scientific studies had proven the correlation between happy and healthy employees and increased revenue. He put the article down and thought back to the scene from the elevator. Eleanor, out of breath, and Angela, rushing by looking stressed and anxious. The twenty something he hadn't even had time to introduce himself to. Don, the middle aged executive he'd known for years, who had probably just returned from a secret smoke break. It was more than just the way they all looked. It was their general energy and emotional and physical well being. It was hard to imagine them representing the company well, when they didn't seem to be taking care of themselves.

John knew that if he adopted a health management program the key would be more than just getting people to sign up. It would mean incentivizing people, but at the right time. He worried about keeping them engaged. It would be an important factor in changing the mindset of the culture. The consultants had gone through it in detail. Engagement had to occur beyond the initial assessment. John walked out to the living room and opened the door to the back porch. His backyard was peaceful and quiet, the manicured grass surrounded by large oak trees. He watched two squirrels give chase up one tree, across the branches, and down the other side. He took a sip of the scotch and just inhaled the fresh air. His thoughts turned back to work and the healthcare program. He finally got it.

In the past he'd been focused on corporate wellness. But now it all clicked in his head. Wellness is about the culture, the support mechanism, and the things the company could do to help people improve. But a health management program would track individual behavior and promote accountability.

The reasons traditional wellness programs did not work was that there was no incentive, no system to track data, and the responsibility fell to the employees desire to participate, versus being driven by the employer. If someone went to the gym or got a preventive checkup, there wasn't any system to track it, follow up, or monitor the data going forward. Without data, there'd be no results.

John thought back to the scene at the elevator. His employees were haggard and rushed. Don, Angela, Eleanor, and the others did not exude health or happiness. If anything, they were the picture of what not to do. They were overweight, unpolished, out of shape, defeated, anxious and stressed. In a nutshell: sick.

I've got a sick culture, he thought. And it's time to make a change.

THREE

Don caught the nine o'clock flight and was in the vendor's plant by noon. As the business development manager for the Northern United States, Don was responsible for managing client and vendor relationships.

The automobile manufacturer had several relationships with vendors that provided various parts and service and it was a challenge to manage them all. Each relationship was different, but they all mattered.

He was responsible for making sure the vendors produced exactly what the market needed, reviewing parts delivery schedules, and cementing critical relationships that would help increase company market share. He would spend the day with the plant manager in meetings with key executives, touring the warehouse, and sitting in on a product development meeting. Then he'd fly home, and get in sometime after midnight.

A large part of his job was to report back on quality standards and objectives, and he was good at it. He knew the company inside and out and had held five positions there over the years, rising through the ranks. He had started on the factory floor, and truly understood the employees and their challenges. But now he sometimes wondered if he had hit a plateau. He hadn't been promoted in four years. He was tired all the time, and couldn't always keep up with the younger employees. In high school he'd been a star running back on the varsity team, but now that seemed like someone else's life. He never worked out, ate pretty poorly, and always felt sluggish. Just getting on the plane and to a business meeting was enough to set him back an entire day.

Don loved his work, but it left him little margin time

for anything else. Visiting the vendors was different than visiting his own company factories because it gave him insight into different cultures, and philosophies. As he stood in the warehouse listening to the plant manager outline a new parts distribution process, his stomach grumbled.

He felt the soreness at the back of his throat that had been lingering for days. He'd had nothing to eat for breakfast but airplane coffee and a stale donut. Just a typical day, he thought. *As soon as this meeting's over I'm getting a burger.* His head pounded, and he lifted his hand to his forehead. At 50, he felt the stress of the fact that his peak earning years were just about peaking.

"Don, you alright?"

The room began spinning. Don felt hot and his palms sweated profusely.

The plant manager looked concerned.

"Do you need water?" a woman asked. "Your face... it's all white."

"I'm fine," he said.

"I think you need to sit down," the woman replied.

Those were the last words he remembered.

A thousand miles away in his hometown, Don's wife Vickie received a phone call from a strange voice. The woman introduced herself as the head nurse of a hospital intensive care unit.

Syracuse? Did the woman say Syracuse? Vickie tried to process the information. Don had traveled to New York on business like he had a million other times. Why would a hospital be calling? It was hard to hear. In the background, the dog barked at a neighbor walking down the street, and music drifted from the television in the living room. She turned it off, and sat down.

"What did you say?" she asked.

"Your husband has been transported to the emergency room," the nurse said. "You should try to get here as soon as possible."

"What? Get where?" The kids were upstairs doing their homework. There was no way she was going anywhere.

"Your husband Don is in the Syracuse General Hospital in Syracuse, New York. He collapsed in a meeting today."

"What?" Vickie couldn't process what the caller was saying.

"You should get the next flight out," the nurse said forcefully. She had been through this before. It would normally take several repetitive sentences before the patients family understood what she was saying. Their first response, was always a numb shock followed by a lot of questions.

"Is he okay? What happened?" Vickie was scared. Her heart clenched.

"He's stable. He's had a cardiovascular event and he's in the Intensive Care Unit."

Vickie choked back tears.

"What's a cardiovascular event?"

"A heart attack," the nurse said.

"Oh my God. I can't believe it." Vickie panicked. Her heart started racing, and the tears flowed.

On the plane to Syracuse the following day, Vickie thought about Don and how he'd taken a flight just a day before, but didn't return. For years he'd taken business trips, with no problem. She knew he was stressed and overweight, but she had nagged him about it until it caused tension between them. Years ago they had walked nightly together, but lately she barely saw him at all. Don was completely wrapped up in his work, and it was killing him. He hardly saw the kids at all, and had missed nearly all of their soccer games. She looked out the airplane window, and her fear turned to anger. How can I raise these kids by myself? She wondered, thinking the worst.

Vickie thought back to all the major milestones in their lives. If she really considered it, she could see that Don had missed most of them trying to achieve, win, and earn. He had spent so much time traveling for work that he'd missed important games, events, graduation ceremonies, and birthday parties. He had felt the pressure to succeed and provide for his family, and it had added a lot of physical and emotional stress to his life. Was it her fault?

She had wanted to be a stay at home mom, so she gave up teaching when their first child was born. She had pressed Don so much about the other moms in their neighborhood who got to stay home until he finally relented and agreed with her. Staying home every day and being there for the kids was the right thing to do. They both agreed to it. But didn't that choice stress them more financially? What if she had retained her teaching career even part time? After all, most days the kids were actually in school for eight hours. So stay at home mom, really meant stay at home, while the kids were now in school every day. It meant that Don worked to support them, traveled, and stressed more about how they'd make ends meet.

Now here she was, at 47 surrounded by business travelers in suits, out of her comfort zone. Truth was, Don wasn't the only one who had grown set in his ways. Vickie hadn't missed a yoga class or a day with the kids in years. She had never traveled alone, and never with Don though he'd invited her. The stress began to build.

The flight attendant passed by and Vickie put her hand up, as if summoning a waitress. "Excuse me!"

The flight attendant wore a navy vest. It was worn, and had decades of pins and patches. Her gold necklaces had charms and crosses, and Vickie guessed her to be about fifty five. Older than Don, and probably the same amount of miles.

The last time Vickie had flown, on their honeymoon, the flight attendants were younger, with long hair and crisp ironed uniforms. What had happened? The attendant gave her a weary smile that said she'd lost her passion for flying years ago.

"Yes?" the flight attendant looked at Vickie impatiently. She scanned the cabin and pushed on the seat back, moving it into its upright position.

"I need a drink," Vickie explained. "You still have those?"

She felt like a cave man leaving her dark corner of the world for the first time.

"Yes, we sell drinks. What can I get you? Pepsi? Mountain Dew? Water?"

Vickie shook her head.

"I'll need something a lot stronger than that. How about Cabernet?"

The flight attendant reached into the cart. "Seven dollars."

Vickie shook her head and reached for her wallet. "That's highway robbery."

"Nothings free," the flight attendant shot back. "Been a rule for a long time now."

"But... I thought I just saw you give that guy over there a small bottle for free..."

Vickie handed the flight attendant a ten dollar bill and the woman reached into the cart for the wine and change.

Vickie poured it, leaned back in her chair, and let the wine singe the back of her throat. It took some of her worries away, and as she stared out the window she thought of her two daughters, and their life together. She couldn't support them without Don. She could go back and renew her teaching license, but on a teacher's salary, how would they pay the mortgage?

They hadn't planned for any of these things.

Her thoughts turned to anger. Why didn't Don go

to the doctor sooner? If he had a disabling disease and was out of work, what kind of life would they have? The questions swirled in her mind. She thought about when they first met, and how they used to jog together on weekends. They had an active life, but it slowed down when Don began working so hard, until it stopped altogether. His old college football pictures were still displayed in the photo album on the coffee table. But Don hadn't been an athlete since he graduated. Even though she had begged him to walk, jog, or bike ride with her, he always said he didn't have time.

When the plane landed in Syracuse, she was feeling numb. By the time she ran through the airport, found a taxi, and got to the hospital, it was dark. She bolted through the emergency room door and found a nurse.

"I need to see my husband!" she shouted. "Don Miller."

The head nurse stood. She wore baby blue scrubs and a name tag that said Penelope. It was the same name as her own grandmother.

"I need to know if he's okay," she demanded.

The nurse touched her arm. "Ma'am, calm down. I understand."

Vickie sobbed. "I need to see my husband!"

The nurse helped her to a chair. She let Vickie cry for

a moment, and then chose her words slowly. "No one expects this. Sadly, I see this every day. People just go about their lives, living and working, and don't expect anything bad to happen."

"He should've listened to me..." Vickie said. "I have been asking him to make changes in his life. To stop neglecting his health..."

"I can bring you upstairs to his room," the nurse said. "But he needs his rest."

Vickie just sat, numb. There were so many things she wanted to say to him. But in some ways she blamed herself. She knew they should have incorporated healthy habits into their life. She knew she could have gotten them all into a morning routine, or an evening walking schedule, or even helped her husband develop healthier eating habits by making healthy meals for dinner. Instead she buckled to his schedule and often ordered pizza, or whatever was most convenient. Most nights they ate separately, and she fed the kids fast food through the drive through on the way to their games or after school activities. Finally, the culmination of all those bad small decisions had added up, resulting in a major life threatening event.

It was hard to believe it had come to this.

FOUR

John pulled into the office building parking garage when he received the call.

Don, his longtime employee, was in a hospital bed in Syracuse. He'd suffered a mild heart attack, and was undergoing testing and care in ICU.

The CEO sat in the car and thought about it for awhile. He had scheduled this morning's meeting with the intention of getting his leadership team interested in implementing the corporate health management program, and he was convinced now more than ever that they needed it. A health management program was the answer to reducing costs and creating a better culture. But could it also save lives?

He wondered, "If I would have implemented the program sooner, would this have happened?"

John thought back to the day he'd first hired Don, when the company was small. Don had kids of his own and they both had a lot in common. Early on they shared dinners together, and John invited Don to golf with him and potential customers, as they forged the future of the company together. Then they began building it, brick by brick, until the distance between them widened. The CEO worked tirelessly and soon months had passed before he saw Don or even his own family, as he went from deal to deal and prospect to prospect, just building. Eventually the company grew. It grew so large that now there were days he hardly recognized anyone in the hallway.

John thought back to the day he first made the decision to start a company. He had started it with an idea, on a cocktail napkin, sitting alone with a beer in an outdoor cafe. He remembered the hope and anticipation of that moment, and how all good things had converged up until then, to create the company he had today. It had seemed as if the people places and things had all fallen into place. The day he opened his doors was a watershed moment. One of the best and most significant days of his life. He knew everyone's name, because they had started with only thirty employees, and then after a year they'd grown to a hundred but still he knew everyone's name. But now over a decade later, he saw people in the hallways that he just didn't recognize. The early time in a business was fun and new and all about celebrating wins. But now he wondered why they had grown so big that they lost sight of the human element. In the past he'd had personal dinners with Don and his wife, and members of the sales team at their homes.

Back then, life was easy and the culture was easy to maintain. But today he had culture coaches, management consultants, and big six firms to teach them about how to win various industry awards and achieve more. Always it was about culture, and achieving more. In some ways they were right. Culture could change an organization, but what happens when you've got 5,000 people?

John thought back to the reason he started his company in the first place. He wanted to break the cycle of the things that had been lacking in his own life, and in some ways, he knew he wanted to prove something to himself. He wanted to prove that he could create something from nothing, and that he could actually build a great company despite his limited training. There were a lot of guys that were smarter, or had more money. Some of them had created and sold multi million dollar corporations from just an idea. He admired those guys. Those were the ones that had an anything is possible mindset.

Today the magnitude of where they were as a culture was impossible to ignore. By the time he got to the boardroom, several members of his management team had gathered around the large conference table. The team included the CFO, and executives from HR, manufacturing, legal, and client services. There was a vacant seat, and it should have been filled by Don.

"As most of you know, Don is not here today," he said somberly. "He's in the hospital in Syracuse New York."

The room erupted in discussion. Many already

knew.

"This is why we are here," he said. "I think it's been clear for a long time that we need to do something to improve health in our company."

"Agreed," said the CFO.

The director of the legal department spoke up. "Let's be careful not to mention the details of what happened to Don to anyone. Privacy is important when it comes to personal medical information."

"Having a vendor actually helps the company and the employees maintain privacy," John said. "It takes us out of the middle of the equation."

"We had this at my former company," said an executive. "They gave us incentives for meeting certain outcomes. It actually worked. They had a process where you could earn credits towards lowering your insurance premium."

The consultant spoke. "Incentives are important for behavioral change. They reward employees individually for completing certain activities such as preventive care checkups. Employees can get credits against their premiums, for instance. Or earn points for doing things, like say, getting a mammogram."

"But what does the company get out of it?" an executive asked, "and is there a way to track it?"

"Healthier employees, and reduced healthcare costs," the CEO answered. "This is why our health benefit consultants are here. They're the experts. They help provide value and expertise on how to navigate the healthcare world."

"And, when you adopt a health management program internally," the consultant said, "we'll help you put a plan and also the right products in place that align with your overall company vision."

"Sounds good to me," said the CEO. "I'm all in."

The consultant spoke up. "And, if you want to know how it affects costs, we can actually track medical claims data on a month-to-month basis to gain a true snapshot of the program's return on investment. Claims are statistically lower for employees who participate."

"I don't want to sound like a downer, but how do you track results?" Judy asked.

"The first way we track results is though participation," the consultant said. "If we set the goal the right way, people will know they have to participate in their preventive care plan in order to reduce their own personal premium costs or earn certain incentives. And then, when we track participation levels we'll be able to understand if we are making an impact on reducing overall claims."

"I like that," said the CFO. "So this company that will be implementing the program. Tell us a bit about what they do. I mean, I get the performance discount for employees, but it seems ironic that we are asking doctors to get paid for how well they perform, and yet the consumer is not asked to step up, take responsibility and "pay" for how they perform."

"That's right," the consultant said, "the average American is overweight, hasn't had preventive care done in years and probably has a chronic condition. Why should the person who doesn't take care of themselves at all, pay the same as someone who does? The healthcare management company will track the performance of people's behaviors to set rates for what they pay for coverage."

"Sounds simple. What's step one?" asked the CEO. "Explain to the team what happens when an employee decides to participate in a program like this."

"In the beginning of the program, every individual

employee completes a personal assessment that gives them their health score. It's a weighted indicator of each employee's overall health; and then from there, the health program can assess personal health risk levels. Then we take that insight and strive to provide the right health advice at the right time and with the right frequency. The nice thing is," the consultant said, "that it's measurable. So the vendor you select to implement your healthcare program will provide a customized solution. They'll provide the tracking and reporting at the corporate level so you can see your reduced healthcare costs over time. But at the employee level, it's all about encouragement and support. That's it at a glance."

The CEO leaned forward at the table. "I would think the benefits outweigh any risks. It seems like it would make us a more attractive employer."

"Yes," the consultant agreed. "The program will track results through a points system. We can determine how participation is going by how points are being earned because employees will earn points through various activities that promote good health."

The CFO looked at the Director of HR. "Judy, how are things going at the plant?"

"Turnover is up this quarter," she said.

"It's up every year," the CEO said. "Why are we having such a hard time attracting people?"

"Long hours, difficult work. It's stressful," Judy replied.

The CEO shook his head. Truth was he hated hearing that about his own company.

He didn't want to drive people to their graves. He wanted to make the company a place where people thrived. A place that supported their lives, not detracted from it.

"What's so stressful? Work should be enjoyable, not stressful. People should be excited to come to work," he said.

Judy thought about it for a moment. She tried to look at it in a different light. Maybe the program could help with retention of employees. Maybe it could help her and her HR team reduce turnover, but also attract new talent. Other companies who had fitness and wellness programs seemed to have positive reputations with prospective job seekers. In fact, she'd lost quite a few employees to companies that provided benefits like that to employees.

"So would you agree that this could help us provide people with even greater benefits?" she asked. "A health management program would send the message that we care about employees," she paused, "I'm just not certain how we will monitor or track it with factory workers. Getting a remote population to participate might be hard."

The consultant interjected. "The health management program vendor will help drive participation. They'll guide you through the steps to get people to engage. And the reason people will participate, is because it's a truly integrated health management package, not just a bunch of one-off activities. The program incentives will be linked back to the bottom line, and they'll provide all the integrated data that will allow you to track things like participation, engagement, cost reductions, and ROI over time."

"I can see problems though," Judy said. "What if someone doesn't want us telling them to be healthier?"

"We aren't mandating health. It's about giving them a choice," said the CFO. "Think about it this way. If you've got a credit score of 750 but someone else has a bad credit score, do you want to be treated equally? You've paid your bills on time, and you should be rewarded for that behavior. Same concept with car insurance.

You're penalized for tickets and pay more, or, you can develop good habits, and pay less for car insurance. Why don't we do that with health insurance?"

"Sounds simple," Judy admitted. "It really does." She thought for a moment. "But we've got remote people in the factories. How will we reach them?"

The consultant smiled. He knew they could reduce costs with the right incentive. "It's all about incentives and driving participation," he answered. "And the process is the same no matter where an employee is located because it's not about one wellness event or a health fair at headquarters. It's customized. Basically we utilize technology to push information to the employee, and they've got the choice to participate, and earn lower healthcare costs, or not. We monitor an individual's behavior and assign a risk index to them."

Judy interrupted. "But we did incentivize them. In the past we gave employees a hundred dollars for completing a questionnaire and another hundred for screening."

"True," said an executive, "but we never had a reason to participate any further."

The consultant walked around the table. " If we give people the right incentive at the wrong time, it won't work. Incentives are about the when."

John was all ears. "What do you mean about the when?"

"Well, there are different ways to incentivize people. There are tangible rewards like iPads, or other gifts, but there are also specific financial rewards when the participant meets certain mile markers. They earn credit towards their health insurance premiums. And the health management program I'm going to recommend has developed a proprietary technology that measures things like participation, so it won't be an unknown. You'll know if employees are engaged.

For instance, we have a client who won't give employees coverage unless they participate in the health management program."

"I'm not sure we are ready for that," the CEO said. "Maybe one day."

"What if we built a program that incentivized them after they've completed their preventive care. So for instance in the past, if you gave someone a hundred dollars for doing a screening you've incentivized them for enrolling in a program. But that's not enough if we want to see risk factor reduction. We want to incentivize them beyond that."

Another consultant from the team spoke up. "Or if they've been diagnosed with a chronic condition and they've actually completed a care plan. Disease management is a big part of cost reduction."

After the meeting was over, John felt as if a big weight had been lifted off of his shoulders. They'd made the decision. The corporate health management program would launch in the weeks to come. They'd promote it internally throughout the quarter, and talk to the program manager about how to drive participation. Participation would be the measuring stick. If they could get a large percentage of their population enrolled, the next step would be to get them engaged.

John walked through the hallway and thought about the demographic of his work force. No matter who they were or what position they held, he felt like they'd like the possibility of saving money on insurance premiums. The program would be a win for everyone, if he could just make them see the value in it.

He turned the corner and stuck his head into Angela's office.

She had been an employee with him since the early days, and had risen through the ranks every couple of years. John knew her personality. She was a doer, and a leader. On top of that, she had an intrinsic desire to make things work, because she not only wanted to make her life better, but also her daughter's. People like that would be easy to engage because they had an internal motivation driving them. But he wondered about the others. Angela would be one of the compliant ones, but the program would need to appeal to the executives, and also the factory workers and mid level employees. Angela would be a great champion to help get the workforce engaged from the inside out.

"Hey, can I chat with you about something?" he asked.

Angela turned in her chair. When she saw him, she stood. "Sure! What's up?"

"I've been thinking a lot about what we do. And what we can do better," he said. He sat down and outlined the health management program, and told her about all the benefits for employees. The ways they could save, the ways they could focus more on getting healthier. He reviewed the program and how employees would get reminders to go to the next preventive step, such as when it was time for their annual physical wellness exam, or mammogram. He told her about the web portal and how all the data would be confidential and stored in one place. Angela listened intently.

"Well?" he asked. "What do you think?"

"Sounds like something we really need," she said.

"We are considering putting a premium credit in place that will incentivize you and all employees for participating in our program, not just enrolling in the program, but also being engaged. You'll need to complete your annual preventive care and based on your health profile, complete the necessary steps to maintain and control your health," John explained, "but if you do these things, you will spend less for coverage. Would you participate in something like that?"

"Absolutely. I've got a daughter, and I pay for both of us. So if I can earn credits towards that premium, I would absolutely participate."

Angela thought about Jessica. Her daughter had gained weight in recent years, and was borderline diabetic. Angela worried about that. She had read the statistics, that thousands of American kids were diagnosed with diabetes simply because of bad choices. But ultimately, those choices for what food to eat or not, come down to the parent. Too many nights Angela chose fast food, or processed foods, instead of going home to prepare a healthy meal with vegetables. In fact, if she thought about it, vegetables were very low on their list of foods. Most of the time she made pasta, or chicken, or whatever they could get on the fly in between school activities. All of it made her feel guilty. What if she was harming the health of her child?

"That's right," John said. "It will save you a lot of money."

Angela sighed. "I'm so out of shape!" she said, laughing uncomfortably. "I need to!"

It was the truth and she knew it.

Besides that she had sleepless nights, anxiety, and days where she just didn't think it was possible to get everything done.

Work had been stressful, and if she didn't get a report or assignment finished on time she'd stay awake nights thinking about it.

She wanted everything to be perfect but she felt as if it rarely was. Sometimes she stayed late after work just together a report done in time for the next days deadline, going over it time and time again. She had always been a perfectionist, sometimes to the point of neglecting relationships. Work projects had to be just right. She didn't want anyone to think she wasn't capable of doing her job. She knew she couldn't be satisfied until it was perfect, but striving for that goal often left her short in other areas. Her daughter Jessica would sometimes have to cook her own dinner, or get a ride home from school.

Angela had been divorced for five years, and in that time frame her daughter had gained weight too, and withdrawn deeper into a life of video games and Cheetos after school. Some days, they barely had time to talk.

"I think I've gained ten pounds just in the last six months with all the traveling that's been required," she told the CEO. But then she wished she could've taken it back. What if he thought she was complaining? What if her job was in jeopardy? She had to do everything possible to keep a stable career and health benefits, at least until her daughter went off to college. These were the fears that kept her up at night. Losing her income and having no insurance.

Angela rubbed her head. She felt swollen and achy, and constantly popped Tums like candy. She was a shadow self of the woman she had been. Yes, she needed a program to get her focused on health!

When she saw the CEO at the elevator the other day she had hardly wanted to stop, for fear he'd ask her a question about the sales numbers. Things were slipping. Clients felt the tension, and some even commented on it. She spent most of her time reacting and repairing these days, it seemed.

"I'd like you to take an active role in this program," John said.

"Sure," Angela replied. "Absolutely. Anything you need."

"I need champions. I need people like you, internally,

who are willing to set the example for the others, lead health initiatives when we have them, and talk up the positive aspects of this program with the employees."

"I'm in," she said. "Sounds great!" Angela felt hopeful because of the new vision. The CEO seemed intent on changing the mindset of the culture from stagnant and overworked, to healthy and well. She felt herself relaxing simply at the thought of being involved in a shift towards health.

On the way back to his office John thought of Don, in the hospital room. He didn't want to see it happen again to anyone else on his team.

The time is now, he thought. It's time to take control.

FIVE

Vickie paced the corridor inhaling the pungent smell of antiseptic and decay. Hospitals smelled like a mixture of bleach, sick people, and cleaning supplies. Her insides objected to the thought of disease and germs all around her.

The nurse asked her to follow her down the brightly lit fluorescent hallway. Vickie wondered, why couldn't hospitals be made to look like hotels? It seemed to make no sense. The place you go to get well looks like a place you'd never choose to go in the first place. Stark, pale walls, sterile furniture and plastic mixed with chrome tables. The hospital had more in common with the funeral home, than a place of life. They took an elevator to the third floor, and stood in awkward silence until the doors opened. Vickie followed the nurse to room 303.

Inside, a tall, lean doctor in a long white lab coat stood beside the bed. Don had his eyes closed, and was connected to monitors via wires and tubes. An IV ran through his left arm, dripping some sort of yellowish fluid.

Vickie couldn't take her eyes off of her husband. Her mind raced with fear and regret. I knew I should've made him go to those doctors appointments, she thought. I knew I should've made him eat better.

The doctor turned and extended a hand. His expression was serious.

"Dr. Stevens," he said sternly. "Please, sit down."

Vickie did as he said and sat in a chair by the edge of the bed. She touched Don's hand and he opened his eyes, and forced a smile.

"How are you?" she asked softly.

"I've been better," Don whispered. His voice sounded raspy and weak.

She turned to the doctor. "What's going on? Is he going to be okay?"

"Ma'am, your husband has had a heart attack," the doctor replied. "I would refer to it as mild, however no heart attack is mild. They're all significant. He may have damage to his kidneys, and does have some permanent damage to his heart. Honestly, he's a very lucky man. When he got here he was a ticking time bomb."

Vickie just sat quietly. She had so many questions.

"Tests show that his numbers are quite frankly off the charts," the doctor continued. His cholesterol is high. His blood pressure is bad. He has had diabetes for a while now but apparently it went undetected. He said he hasn't had a physical in three years. Is that right?"

Vickie nodded. "Maybe longer than that. I scheduled several doctors appointments and I don't think he made it to even one of them. The last one he canceled because of a business trip."

The doctor looked down at Don. "You can't earn money for your family if you're dead," he said bluntly. "You've got to stop putting your health second."

Don closed his eyes. "I know."

"No, you don't know. If you'd listened to me we

wouldn't be in this mess," Vickie interrupted.

"I've got a mortgage to pay," Don whispered.

No one said anything for a long time. The machines hummed. One made a beeping sound, and the image on the screen spiked. The doctor put his stethoscope against Don' chest.

"He's got to stop smoking," the doctor said.

"He doesn't smoke," Vickie replied.

The doctor narrowed his eyes at Don, but moved on. It wasn't uncommon for a patient to hide things from their families. But negative health habits always made their way to the surface sooner or later.

Don didn't say anything. He knew it wasn't the time to come out with an all out confession about the ways he'd been harming his health and his family. He had said he'd given up smoking years ago, but the truth was he never did. He just hid it well, and smoked at work or on the way home.

"There are other ways to cope with stress," the doctor said. Much of what your husband is experiencing is the result of stress."

"What do you mean?" Vickie asked, worried.

"Stress causes poor choices, and decisions to cover up the stress. Those bad decisions just make the situation worse and it becomes a compound effect of negative choices and outcomes. Everything originates from stress. Mental stress is the cause of most disease whether we realize it or not. When there's financial stress, people work more and they neglect their health. They tend to overeat. At the root of diabetes, obesity, cardiovascular disease is stress that has been ignored."

Don took a deep breath, but said nothing.

"What's next?" his wife asked.

The doctor smiled. "Well, it's not too late. He's alive. And now is the time to make the changes that will impact the rest of your life."

Don listened quietly. He couldn't believe he was listening to others talk about his health and his life as if he were a little kid in the principal's office. He felt disempowered. Like a failure, instead of the leader of his family.

If he had to admit it, the truth was he had neglected his health. No one took it away from him. He knew he had made the choice to work harder, and make more money, each day all while ignoring the chest pains he'd been having. They would come and go, and they weren't really that bad but he knew deep inside that they were a warning sign. He should have chosen better meals. He should have taken the stairs or jogged every morning in the hotel on business trips. Instead he chose room service, eggs Benedict, and surfing the net before his business meetings in the morning. Most of all, Don knew he should have kept the doctors appointments and gotten preventive bloodwork done. Maybe his diabetes would've been diagnosed much sooner.

"We have to keep him in the hospital at least a few more days," the doctor said. "Your husband is about thirty pounds overweight. Right now he's got the body of a man twenty years older. He's going to have to make some radical lifestyle changes."

Don couldn't believe what he was hearing. It was all so surreal.

"Why do you have to keep him so long?" Vickie asked.

"This isn't an overnight solution" the doctor said. "It's taken years of bad habits to get to this point." He looked down at Don.

"Now is a good time to try to figure out what's causing all this build up of stress in your life so that we can help you find solutions to change it. We've got nutritionists and mental health specialists who are available to meet with you while you're here to offer you some options."

Don nodded. Seemed painless.

"What are you so stressed about?" Vickie asked.

"We have a simple life."

Don shook his head. "Simple?" he felt defeated.

"We have a great family. You've got a good job..."

"Bills," he said.

"Well, everyone's got bills," Vickie said. "It's a part of life."

"Every month more bills arrive," Don said, exasperated, "and we have two kids about to enter college, and a mortgage and two car payments. I'm pushing fifty-five, Vickie. How long do you think I'm going to be able to support our family and meet all of our needs?"

Vickie just sat, stunned. She'd never heard him talk like this before.

"We've got a lot of financial stress. It's been weighing on my mind. We've got a big house. A big life. I just don't know how we're going to do it all. I work overtime to try to reach my numbers so I can get my annual bonus. It's a lot for one person to deal with. I know I don't eat right when I travel or work late at the office. There's just no time. And, I've been smoking again. I have not been making good choices."

"And drinking a lot more," Vickie added.

"All of those things help take the pressure off," Don admitted.

"In the short term," the doctor said, interrupting. "But they end up compounding your stress. Especially when they lead to physical problems."

"I can go back to teaching," Vickie said. "There are other solutions to bring in more money."

The doctor checked his watch. "These are all good things for you to talk about as a family. Honestly, I see a lot of families in here who don't get that same opportunity. The good news is that your health is in your own hands. It's not too late to turn it around."

SIX

The CEO jogged up the stairs in the morning, and passed the posters promoting the health fair screening event. The new health management program had been implemented, and the company they'd selected had already delivered more than promised.

Everything he had orchestrated behind the scenes with his own team, such as the health care program objectives, implementation strategy, and mission statement that would be communicated to employees, had been executed. His team had met with the vendor to outline specifics of how they'd communicate the program, and what the platform would be. Even before the program went live, they structured it in a way that would be easily embraced and communicated. And the response was overwhelmingly positive!

John was most surprised by how much his own life had shifted. His mood was light, and the stress had dissipated. Now, he was looking forward to the employee screening day on campus. Hundreds of employees had already signed up to attend.

The event would be the beginning of a new era for the company. The cafeteria would be converted into a health screening event, with basic testing equipment and health experts on-site. Employees would spend private, one-on-one time with a screening specialist and get their individual biometric screening. The short health examination would test height and weight, waist circumference, blood pressure, blood glucose and lipid profile. The lipid profile, a blood test that measures HDL, LDL, Total Cholesterol, Triglycerides, and a cardiac-risk ratio, would help determine a baseline of health.

Angela turned away from the elevator in the lobby of her office building, where a crowd of suits stood. A poster on the wall beside the elevator showed an image of a girl in running shorts and sneakers, stretching.

The caption read: *Be strong. The time is now.*

The message inspired her.

Today is the day I take back my life, she thought.

Angela walked down the long corridor, and passed other inspiring posters with similar messages.

Live your dream. Be healthy, balanced, and inspired.

One jumped off of the wall at her.

The time is now!

Angela found the door to the stairwell.

In an instant she flung the door open and sprinted up the stairs; her mind almost as elevated as her heart. By the time she reached her desk she felt energized! It was as if all of the dormant nerves and muscles had kicked in to gear at once, remembering what it was like to be active again.

Back at her desk she felt a rush inside, a kind of endorphin high. Her eyes scanned the beige walls, overlooking all the accolades of the sales team's success. Every accomplishment in a frame was work related, except one. Her focus landed on a small frame containing a race number and medal from five years ago.

Rocky Mountain Marathon. Her heart sank. Now she couldn't run a mile if she tried. The words from the posters rang in her head. Be strong. The time is now!

Angela logged on to the health management portal. She read a message that outlined an incentive program for getting fit, and how to be eligible to earn a lower premium. Just like the CEO had said, the company would be providing rewards for fitness, eating healthier, and getting preventive testing.

Step one was to complete an online assessment, and she'd done that.

In less than fifteen minutes she had completed it and it had prompted her through basic health and lifestyle questions.

Did she smoke? No. Exercise? Not enough. Drink? Just a glass of wine, occasionally. After the assessment she browsed through the online portal and read more of the information there. Next step would be to participate in the onsite screening event that day, and then review the results with a health coach.

Angela navigated through the portal for a few minutes, reading information and health tips about diet and exercise. She printed out some information about changes she could make.

The time is now, she thought. Today is the day I make a positive change.

The biggest motivation for participating in the health management program was the incentives. She started downstairs, for the health screening event.

The CEO wanted to set a good example, and walk the talk. So he headed back down to the screening event just before it started, and was the first one in line.

Angela showed up a minute later.

"Hey!" he said, somewhat surprised.

"What, you didn't think I'd participate?" Angela laughed. "I told you I would! I was hoping to be first in line."

John smiled. Other employees streamed in slowly, and stood in line. John got his blood pressure, and other vital signs checked first.

"A normal blood pressure should be between 120 over 80 to 140 over 90," the specialist said. "Your's is a bit high."

"Really?" the CEO was surprised.

"It should be within this range." the specialist pointed to a chart. "But it's elevated."

The specialist explained it in greater detail. John was borderline at risk, and his cholesterol was also borderline.

John headed back to his office, thinking about the results. He was astounded actually, and couldn't get it out of his mind. He knew some of his employees would have health issues, but he never thought he'd have any unusual test results. It surprised him. He closed the door to his office and sat down at the computer. He filled out the health risk assessment, and realized that for the very first time he was analyzing his own health, stress levels, his nutrition habits (or lack thereof) and how active (or inactive) he really was. Here he was, CEO of a company, yet overlooking the one thing that was most important - his overall wellness. John sat back in his chair, and exhaled. It was a pivotal moment, and it opened his eyes. Not only did his culture need to be awakened, but he did too. He'd neglected his preventive care, and had focused too much on work, over his health. But he was determined to turn things around.

John called and left a message for the doctor to schedule his annual checkup.

After just a few weeks he already felt healthier, stronger, and more mentally clear. He invited one of his top corporate clients to participate in his company's 5k, and started sending out personal weekly emails to his employees to encourage participation in the corporate health management program. For the first time he felt like he was leading. Not just reacting, but leading the mission towards a healthier, happier culture. Now he was seeing employees walk the stairs again instead of taking the elevator. And in the lunchroom, they were discussing menu items, and making healthier choices, because the experts from their health management company had brought in a dietician to look over the menu. Now, the employees had truly nutritious choices, not just fast food. It was almost as if they'd been given permission to be healthy.

On Monday, he passed through the cubicles on the seventh floor on the way to his office and instead of taking the shortcut, he stopped in the break room where a handful of employees had congregated. The health management company they'd hired had encouraged him to support the program through actively participating himself, and communicating to his employees. In addition to the weekly communication the CEO sent to his team, he decided to spend more time encouraging employees face to face. He stopped and chatted for awhile. Then he continued on walking through the halls, and stopping in cubicles.

He passed by Angela's office and saw her sitting at her desk on a large red workout ball while she worked at her computer. Her whole mood seemed lighter than the last time he'd seen her.

"You going to join me in the company 5k?" he asked.

Angela turned and smiled. She showed him her electronic calendar. It's right there, see?" The date was highlighted. "I just started training."

"Great job. Take people with you!"

"I invited a few people already," she said.

He looked at the quote she had taped to her computer.

Today is the day, I make a different choice. The time is now!

SEVEN

In the weeks that followed the screening, the people Angela talked to in the health management program had been reassuring and emphasized that change was truly possible. They offered her ongoing access to her health coach who was available through the company's online web portal and by phone.

Angela had learned during the screening that her cholesterol was high, which really didn't surprise her.

She loved cheese, and other foods that elevated cholesterol. Plus, it was hereditary. Her mom had high cholesterol.

When Jeff the health coach first called, they talked
about how to lower it to a healthy number and he offered Angela several specific solutions, including regular exercise and a diet low in fat and full of fruits and
vegetables. He also advised Angela to go for a more in
depth physical, something she hadn't done in years.
She'd need her well woman exam, a mammogram, and
a basic evaluation.

"Have you had your preventive care?" Jeff asked.
"Because that's important."

Angela loved how her coach was professional, yet
persistent. He encouraged her to get her preventive
care, without pushing.

They had talked three times, and already she felt as if
she had a trusted advisor who was guiding her through
her own individual customized health and fitness plan.

On Friday morning Angela returned a voicemail
from Jeff, her coach.

"It's Angela," she said. "I figured what better way to
start my day than to talk to you."

Jeff pulled up her electronic file. "Hi Angela, how are
you?"

He could see that she had already completed her

health assessment, and her biometric screening. She had received her Health Score, which would be the basis of knowledge for going forward. The Health Score was the result of a combination of individual variables, based on a combination of answers to the questions asked in the Member Health Assessment and the Biometric Screening results. A high Health Score could indicate that health decisions and current health status are on the right track. A low Health Score suggested that someone could be at a greater risk of developing certain diseases and health problems.

Now that she knew her risk factors, she was in the action phase of the corporate health management plan. He would encourage her to browse the online portal and engage with the health management system to learn more.

"It's been great for me," Angela admitted. "I'm motivated to succeed now that there are financial incentives tied to my behavior. It's actually helping me develop better habits. Before, I just worked all the time. Now I've got an incentive to stay in shape."

Each day she looked at her calendar and logged her calories. It was one of the things her coach had advised her to do. Count her calories, and stay within her daily limit to keep her weight under control.

The coach was pleased she had made it a priority. He had no doubt she would succeed. Angela would be one of his success stories.

Later that week Angela decided to skip her regular sit down lunch in the cafeteria, and had an apple and a hardboiled egg instead, so she could take a walk. It was a nice change, and she felt more energized than ever. Each day she had chatted with her colleagues who had formed a morning running club to train for the 5k. She considered joining them, and also made a mental note to get her daughter involved by training with her after school. She was only 12, but wasn't it time to set a good example for her?

She didn't want Jessica to end up a workaholic like she'd been the past few years. She was beginning to wonder if her own hectic lifestyle and neglect of her health had shaped her daughter's self-esteem. Jessica never did anything physical, and her confidence suffered because of the extra weight. If she'd played soccer, or had been in cheerleading, Angela wondered, would it have been different? Organized sports could have helped her grow and develop as a person. And excelling athletically would've built her self-esteem and benefited her health at the same time.

The school nurse had sent home some papers a year

ago warning Angela to focus on giving her daughter healthy foods, because Jessica had been in the nurse's office three times during physical education class, for nausea. Truth was, she couldn't even jog the mile required for her grade, so the nurse let her come sit with her when she felt sick. Angela was regretful when she thought back to those conversations. Now it was difficult to see what a year of fast food and busy lives had done. Jessica had low self-esteem, and it was hard to watch her lose confidence, and withdraw more into herself.

Angela vowed to turn things around for both of them. And her company supported the process by providing the tools and resources to help make the necessary changes that would impact her health for a lifetime. If she met all her requirements, she'd even get paid back.

When she got home that night, she made a low fat chicken salad for the two of them, and then handed Jessica a box.

"What's this?" her daughter asked.

"I stopped at the sports store on the way home and got you a new pair of running shoes. It's their latest style."

Jessica tore into the box and pulled out a pair of pink and yellow running shoes. "I love them!" She immediately tried them on.

Angela smiled. She knew from her employers' health management program that incentives worked. She had earned financial incentives for meeting all her basic goals, and now she knew there were more on the road ahead. Incentives worked, so she'd use the same principle at home.

"Want to go for a jog?" she said.

Her daughter smiled and laced up the shoes. "Yes!"

EIGHT

On Monday Angela laced up and walked briskly up the eleven flights of stairs to her office, just to see if she could. At the top step she waited in the stairwell, out of breath, gasping. She stood for awhile until her heart rate came down and walked out the door to the hallway into the offices, feeling empowered. What if I did that each and every day? she wondered. One simple addition that didn't take more than ten minutes. Instead of the elevator, she'd wear her running shoes to the office in the morning and challenge the stairs. Already she felt stronger.

In her office she immediately went online and spent time looking through her health scores on the wellness portal. There were a lot of things she needed to work on, but she also found lots of educational resources with tips on how to make lifestyle changes that lead to results. She decided to take a nutritional webinar to address her diet, and earn points towards her incentive. The webinar was facilitated by a registered dietician and was only 15 minutes long. She learned about fats and sodium and found that she actually enjoyed learning about nutrition.

Once it was over, a text came from her colleague, Eleanor.

Let's meet in the café, it's the Italian buffet today. They've got that great lasagna!

Angela text back.

I'm sorry, I can't. I'm committed to getting active everyday at lunch time.

As soon as she sent the text, she was proud of herself. She knew that avoiding the big lunches would be her biggest obstacle. She enjoyed the time with friends, chatting about the workday. And, she loved the cheese-cake. But getting fit would be a series of small choices, each and everyday. A compound effect that added up. Eleanor was about sixty pounds overweight, and Angela noticed how she herself had packed on the pounds just by hanging out with her for a few months. A text came back.

You serious?

Yes. Angela replied.

Angela woke up the next day after her first few weeks of work, working out, and making healthier choices, feeling more alive than she had in months. It was a whole new schedule. Work, work out, eat right. Work, work out, eat right. It was so simple.

She took the stairs instead of the elevator, and when she got to her desk she saw a group of women gathered around her coworker's office having coffee and sharing stories. A box of creme filled donuts sat on the table. Instantly, she wanted one. Angela walked over. "Good morning girls!"

Eleanor held a donut and a coffee. "Good morning! Want a donut?"

Angela hesitated. She knew if she stayed too long that she'd succumb to the temptation for sweets. "No way," she said. "I'm training for a 5k."

"You only live once," someone said.

"Yeah, plus, you can always skip dinner. The donut is worth it," said another.

"Okay fine," she said, taking one.

Angela ate it in less than a minute as she walked back to her office. When it was done she threw the napkin in the wastebasket under her desk and immediately felt disappointed. And that was the cycle. Spontaneous decisions, and then regret. She thought about her divorce and everything leading up to it. Decisions, and then regret. Angela started to feel depressed about the whole thing. What if she couldn't make any lasting change? What if she was destined to gain ten pounds every couple of years until she couldn't get it off? What if she never got married again because men found her unattractive? The questions just compounded in her mind.

She'd done so well the past few weeks. It was a small setback, but when she added that to the wine she'd had on the girls night out last Friday, she wondered if she could ever make it up. All those excess calories would prevent her from losing the weight she wanted to, to get to her goal. Eight or ten pounds was a hard goal and she knew that she would have to be disciplined each and every day to do it. Each time she compromised, she felt bad about it. It's so stupid, she thought, feeling bad about a dumb donut. But inside, it wasn't the donut that bothered her, but the fact that she had taken a step back. She felt like a failure. Like she'd failed her daughter, and herself. Angela called Jeff, the wellness coach. She explained how she was feeling. He listened to her patiently. "I feel like a failure!" She said.

"Well, I understand…" Jeff replied, "but honestly I think you're being too hard on yourself."

"Really?" She exhaled a big sigh of relief.

"It's about progress, not perfection," he said. "Stay the course and make better decisions everyday. You can do this Angela."

When she hung up Angela felt encouraged. Jeff had given her a different viewpoint, and helped her see that things weren't going to change overnight. She didn't have to be so hard on herself! She went online and spent time looking through the wellness portal. There were a lot of things she needed to work on. But she also found lots of educational resources with tips on how to make lifestyle changes that lead to results. Just taking that one small step made her feel a little bit better. Stop being so hard on yourself, she thought. It's only a donut. - change to "When she hung up Angela felt encouraged. Jeff had given her a different viewpoint, and helped her see that things weren't going to change overnight. She didn't have to be so hard on herself! She went online and spent time looking through resources with tips on how to make lifestyle changes that lead to results. Just tak- ing that one small step made her feel a little bit better. Stop being so hard on yourself, she thought. It's only a donut.

She thought about Don, her coworker, and sent him a quick email. Hope you're back with us soon, she said. If you need anything at all let us know.

In the small hospital bed thousands of miles away, Don's mind swirled with thoughts. The food was cold, the room was colder, and the thin blanket barely covered his body. Back home, he envisioned Vickie under the down comforter they'd bought at Nordstrom's when they got their first house. He remembered it because it was the first time they'd spent more than two hundred dollars on just a blanket, and he'd worked hard for it. Now he couldn't help but reflect on his life. Here I am, he thought, wasting away in this cold hospital bed eating boxed mashed potatoes, with the smell of antiseptic all around me. Back home, Vickie and the kids would make French toast or scrambled eggs with cheese, or whatever it was they made for breakfast these days. And they'll be sleeping under a warm blanket at night, he thought.

He felt powerless, and began wondering if he'd ever

be able to go back to work again. What if this is it? He thought about the stories he'd heard about men who went to the hospital and got some crazy infection, and never went home. One question after another came like rapid fire. What if there's something worse wrong with me? What if I lose my clients? He thought about his job, and worry set in. With the end of the quarter goals coming up it would be hard to reach his numbers, if he took any time off. As it was, he had to spend time visiting vendors, dealerships, and cementing partnerships.

The up-and-coming executive on the West Coast was always after his clients. What if they let him have my accounts? Don started to worry more, and it made his heart hurt. He felt it racing, and his entire body got warmer. He began to worry again, about money, his house, and his accounts. Don envisioned his colleague in his top client's office, and how the client would probably enjoy talking to him about fitness, one of her passions.

His competitor was in his late thirties, and at least ten pounds thinner. A marathon runner, Bob was always talking about the latest running shoe or some other thing that made Don tune out. The fears began to creep in. Don felt his heart begin to race, with the stressful thoughts.

And in a pattern he hardly noticed, the fear began to choke him with one toxic thought leading to another, and then another in a downward spiral. What if I lose my job? He thought. What if I lose my house to foreclosure? What if I can't afford to support my wife in the lifestyle she's accustomed to? The questions fired in his mind. Don's heart raced, and he tried to focus on solutions. He decided to turn his thoughts to his health, to the one thing he could control at the moment. He had heard for years that health was a matter of positive daily choices. But he hadn't made those choices, and he had ignored the well meaning advice of others. Now he was paying for it.

Maybe everyone else was on to something, and he really did need to stop and reevaluate his decisions. Everyone else was getting healthier, while he was laid up in the hospital bed.

As he thought back on things now he wondered, what could he have done differently?

NINE

Most days Angela looked forward to working out. She'd joined the company running club and much to her surprise it wasn't as hard as she thought. It was more jogging than running, and soon she found herself looking forward to meeting everyone in the parking lot Monday mornings. On some days, Jessica would join them before school.

By two o'clock each Angela she was dragging, lacking energy. Maybe it was all the working out, or maybe the way she was eating, but she knew she'd talk with her health coach about it. It felt good to have someone to go to for answers. Would he tell her to eat differently? To take in more protein at breakfast, and eat less carbs and snacks during the day? Or would he tell her to get her blood tested? Angela thought through the various conversations they'd have, and looked forward to it.

Either way the positive changes she already made had outweighed anything else, and she'd lost six pounds! Jessica had lost even more.

At school Jessica was being complimented by classmates and teachers. Everyone had noticed the change, and even her grades were improving. Jessica had gained a lot more self confidence, and seemed to embrace new challenges.

On a Friday Angela walked downstairs to the cafeteria for a bottle of water, and saw another poster about a company health screening event. Prior to the company's implementation of the health management plan, she would have avoided it like the plague. But now it seemed interesting to her. She was genuinely interested in learning more, and bringing home that knowledge to Jessica.

When Angela found out that the program was offering reductions in health care premiums for earning a certain number of points, she was happy to learn that she had already earned lots of points for things she had already done and became even more motivated to succeed.

The flyer on the company bulletin board mentioned fitness coaches and education about reducing stress, a nutritionist, life coach, and a book signing by a well known health author.

Angela saw Eleanor standing by an employee manned booth, signing her name to a sign up sheet.

"What did you just sign up for?" Angela asked, laughing.

"It's the company 5k." Eleanor replied.

Angela smiled. "You're going to do it?"

"You bet!" Eleanor said, beaming. "You inspired me."

"When do we start training?" Angela asked.

"Well," Eleanor laughed. "Let's not get crazy. I've got to walk, before I can run."

Judy from HR walked over. "I want in!"

"Then let's start walking and maybe even jogging before work," Angela said.

A man at the booth introduced himself. "Jeff," he

said. "I'm your health coach."

Angela shook his hand. "Nice to finally meet you face to face! How are you?" They had talked on the phone. Jeff was tall, strong, and confident. Exactly as Angela had imagined him. She knew he had a degree in health sciences and a masters degree, too, but she was surprised to see him onsite.

"I've just got to tell you," Eleanor said, "I feel so much less stressed since we started this program. It has been great having someone help map out a plan for me to follow. Not only am I getting the exercise I need, I'm also saving money. And, I really feel like I'm a part of something."

A group of employees gathered at the booth. The CEO had been right. The one thing driving participation the most were incentives, and also accountability.

"It's been great for me too," a girl said.

Angela had seen her once or twice walking the sidewalks during lunch time, and participating in the two minute drill every day. The two minute drill was a new activity the healthcare company had implemented that got everyone on their feet and moving at their desks, or wherever they were.

"I love the two minute drills," Angela said. "I can't

be stressed over a project or hunched over an email if I'm doing jumping jacks. Just doing that for two minutes gets my blood rushing through my body."

"I take those two minutes to stretch," Eleanor said. "I think I'm getting more flexible."

"The drill is a great reminder to move our bodies," Jeff said, "and it's a stress reliever. If we understand stress, and what triggers it in our individual lives, than we can find small and yet instant ways to reduce and eliminate it. That's a big part of a corporate wellness program that works."

"I want you to be my coach!" Eleanor said.

She thought back to the day she was out of breath at the elevator, in front of employees. It had been such an embarrassing moment that it was a turning point in her mind. The entire culture of the company was becoming youthful and energetic, yet here she had been gasping for breath, barely able to take a step. It had been a bit of a wake up call.

Angela thought about her coworker Don again and how she wished he could be there to hear this. Don had paid the price for unhealthy choices. But it wasn't too late for any of them to make a change.

"Making good food decisions will also reduce stress," Jeff said. "Of course doctors know that healthy eating prevents disease, and increases life expectancy. So if you eat healthier, you'll live a longer more vibrant life, and reduce your medical expenses. If you don't have to worry about your health, your life is better."

Angela looked around. Everyone listened intently.

"Just a few generations ago," Jeff continued, "life expectancy was 10 to 15 years shorter on average than it is today. Why? For the same reason everyone smoked. There was a general lack of education about healthy choices and foods."

"I remember the 70's," Eleanor said, "when the advertisements showed good looking, elegant women smoking cigarettes. And the Marlboro man was the icon of handsomeness. Beauty and smoking went hand in hand."

"Today, the advertisements about smoking show real life victims of throat cancer patients with tracheotomies talking in a hoarse voice about why you shouldn't smoke," Angela said matter of factly.

"Today we are a far more open, educated culture," the coach said. "But all we can do is educate people to make better choices."

"It amazes me how many people still smoke," Judy

added.

"In the end it's still up to you. It's a choice each day to make positive changes that will help you live better."

Angela woke up the next morning and immediately put on her running shoes and laced them up. Normally she'd have three cups of coffee and ease into the day. But this time, she vowed to change up everything about her routine. The health management program incentivized her to work harder, and reach all the milestones. It's time to get out of my comfort zone, she thought.

She had done that, and she felt proud of herself. A year ago, she'd sleep through the alarm and barely make it to work on time. But today, she was committed to change. She got up, and laced up her sneakers right away.

Now every week she planned out her meals, and she bought more fresh fruits and vegetables. She and her daughter ate at home more and ate less fast food.

The following morning Jessica came running into the bathroom, frantic.

"Mom! I forgot my homework!"

Angela paused.

"Again?" she could feel the stress and frustration

creep in.

Why was it always this way when they were pressed for time?

She had to get ready for work, get Jessica to school, workout, and get her presentation finished before 10 a.m. and into her boss's office.

"Mom, it'll affect my grade if I don't bring in my homework!"

Helping her daughter with her homework would take up the next hour, at least. She'd miss her workout, and both might be late. She looked at her daughter, exasperated. It was time to stand firm. Healthy habits created healthy bodies. It was what the health coach had taught her.

"I can't help," she said. "I can't bail you out this time. I made a commitment to meet a coworker for a jog."

"Mom!" Jessica pleaded.

"Jessica, I'm sorry. But you've got to start doing your homework when it's due. This is a hard lesson to learn but you need it your entire life. It's about discipline."

Angela knew she wouldn't have said that a few weeks ago. But now, she realized that life was a series of daily choices. She packed her office clothes in a bag for work, so she could change after the workout.

Eleanor will probably cancel, she thought.

When the cell rang on the way to work, she knew who it was.

Eleanor sounded sleepy. Angela envisioned her at home in bed, finding it difficult to get moving.

"I"m driving to work," Angela said. "To meet you. Did you forget our morning run?"

"No, I didn't forget. I'm waiting for you," Eleanor replied. "I got here early so I could stretch before we got started. There are five people here already!"

Angela was surprised. "Really?"

"Yes," Eleanor said, excited. She sounded a bit out of breath. "And can I read you something while you're driving?"

"Sure," Angela said. She heard the rustling of papers on the other end of the line.

"I just got this email last night. Let me read it to you. "It says there's a medical premium reduction for participating in the corporate healthcare program. Did you know that?"

"I did." Angela replied. Eleanor had an accounting degree, so Angela guessed that kind of thing was important to her. "And it also says you can win merchandise, debit cards, or cash incentives," Eleanor said.

Angela turned the car into the company parking lot and saw Eleanor and the others standing there in sneakers and sweatpants. John was there warming up, and chatting with employees. Angela wasn't surprised. She knew he was committed and determined. Each day the CEO had run in the center of the pack, though Angela knew he could break away at any time. Like her, he used to run marathons. He'd joined the employee running club out of obligation, but as it turned out, he actually liked it. Now he looked forward to the hour each morning, and he felt stronger than ever.

The simple act of incorporating movement back into his life, changed everything. Angela could see that he felt stronger, more vibrant, and alive.

John authentically valued the time with his employees, and they could all see it. Instead of being stressed, he laughed and joked with employees. Each week the group grew larger in number. There were about fifty in all, and sometimes they stood around drinking from a giant cooler of Gatorade after the jog. He said it reminded him of his college days when he played soccer, standing around in a parking lot covered in sweat talking about the game.

After just a few weeks in the program Eleanor already looked less stressed, more vibrant, and energized, as if making the decision in her mind had been a domino effect in her body and soul. Angela noticed a difference in Eleanor. She seemed transformed, healthier, and even looked years younger. The program was much more to her than just a health program. Eleanor had saved money on her insurance premium. She stood there in the parking lot, transformed from an out of breath, overworked grandmother just struggling to survive in the corporate world, to a happy, inspired athlete. She beamed.

As if it were the first day, the beginning of the rest of her life.

TEN

Don was released from the hospital on Wednesday and worked all throughout the weekend. On Monday he walked in to find that the employees had decorated his office with banners and signs, and three floral arrangements stood in vases on his desk. One from sales, one from service, and another from a client. It was a nice gesture but Don moved them aside, a bit irritated by the embarrassment of all the attention simply because he'd been unhealthy. He wanted to forget about it all and get back to work.

"Did somebody die?" he said sarcastically. "Looks like a funeral in here!"

"Thankfully it's just a welcome back," Eleanor said, "and not a funeral."

Don opened up email and spent the first hour reviewing the messages. There were welcome back messages from colleagues, and old messages from clients. When he was done with that, he started reviewing client contracts and paperwork. At lunchtime he headed for the cafeteria, and noticed that things looked different in the hallways. There were posters on the wall about a health management program. When he read through it he could see that it offered incentives on his insurance premium for getting healthy.

Don took the elevator downstairs and ordered a slice of pizza from the cafeteria. He decided to take the stairs back up to his office instead, as a compromise for eating bad. He opened the door to the cold stairwell and climbed slowly, stopping at each floor to catch his breath. The words of the doctor rang in his head. Take the stairs, the doctor had said. Walk or jog, instead of taking the elevator.

He thought back to the years past, at their annual conference. In the hotel in the morning after the meetings, he remembered how everyone stood in the lobby in shorts and sneakers. Even Eleanor, the heavy-set administrative assistant, had been there. She wasn't fit, but she wanted to be a team player. Don on the other hand, never felt the desire. Working out had never been his thing.

As he looked around at the posters and new signs reminding him to engage in the corporate health management program, he thought about how reckless he'd been with his own physical health. All those times he hadn't worked out when he had the chance to. Decades of fast food, despite how his wife tried to push him towards healthier choices. Traveling with lots of time in hotel rooms, but making the decision to watch television instead of going to the gym at the hotel. He had neglected his health completely, and now it felt like it was too late. He felt like it was just too far to go to get back up. He knew he needed to lose weight, but he felt embarrassed just at the thought of a doctor telling him to. In all honesty, he never wanted to see a hospital again.

Later that day, he ran into two of his colleagues on the way down to the parking lot. Angela and Bob walked up, and Angela gave him a big hug. Bob asked him how he felt.

"I'm okay," Don said.

"Welcome back," said Bob.

"Thanks guys."

Don was a bit hesitant at what he'd face returning to work, but he had to admit it felt good to have people concerned about him.

"You know we've got a new corporate health management program now?" Bob said. "It might help you with your recovery."

Don said nothing. Truth was, he was on the fence about signing up. He knew that he should, but he hadn't made the decision to enrol yet had a lot of questions.

"I'm glad the company cares enough to support our health," Angela said. "I'm losing weight and I feel better than ever!"

"They give you incentives just for signing up," Bob added.

"And I heard you get a credit on healthcare coverage," Don said. "Is that right?"

Don reached into his briefcase for his medication as they walked.

He found a water fountain and stopped to swallow a blood pressure pill and a cholesterol pill. It gave him a moment to catch his breath. Is this the new life I'm going to live, he wondered? Taking meds and barely keeping up with coworkers on a walk down the hall? Inside, he felt defeated.

That night he told Vickie about the program.

"Perfect timing!" She said, enthused.

The following day, Don's phone rang. He answered, thinking it was his client. But it was Jeff, the corporate health coach.

"Wow, you've been hard to get a hold of," Jeff said. "How are you doing?"

"I've been on vacation," Don said sarcastically. "I got your message about the health screening."

"Well, welcome back," Jeff said. "I wanted to take a few moments to introduce myself and talk through your health management program. Do you have a few minutes?"

"Yep."

"Okay then. Well, please know that everything we talk about on our calls are confidential and private."

"Sounds good," Don said.

Don listened, but he felt that somehow, he wasn't like everyone else.

All around him his colleagues talked about their goals, business, and health management changes. For the most part, he agreed with what they had propositioned about the program, but he was hesitant about change. He thought about the events in his life on the road ahead. His daughter would be getting married in the future, and he wasn't quite sure he was prepared financially or emotionally. It was a different season altogether. Now that he'd gotten them through grade school, maybe it was time to slow down.

"I just wanted to remind you," Jeff said. "Your company rewards you with benefits for getting your preventive checkups. A simple health screening can—and often does—save someone's life. Just learning you've got high blood pressure can save you from potential heart attack or stroke. And diagnosing cancer before it's gotten out of control means you have time to treat it and eliminate it."

"Or," Don interrupted, "you can be like me and fall over in a client warehouse with clogged arteries."

The line was silent. "Sorry to hear that," Jeff said sympathetically. "Are you okay?"

"I suppose," Don said. "I'm back to work."

"Well, truth is, it's good to know what's going on in your body before something goes haywire. And most diseases are treatable. Prevention and management of disease leads to longevity."

"Okay. I've got about seven minutes between calls," Don said. "Tell me what this program is all about. Why do they push those tests? Seems like an invasion of privacy."

"You're actually part of a company that really cares about its employees," Jeff said. "People spend the majority of their time at work, so they figure that's the best place to get healthy and educate people about health. Imagine how healthy our country would be if every company did that."

"Who has time to change habits we've built up our whole life?" Don argued. Inside, he knew it was the right thing for him to do. He needed accountability.

"Behavior is changed over time. If you want to be healthier long term, you have to change your lifestyle today. It's a daily decision."

"Honestly I don't have time to work out at work or anywhere else. When I'm at work, I work," Don said. "There aren't enough hours in the day."

"I understand," Jeff said.

He thought about how everyone else he'd talked to had been genuinely motivated by the program, not only the cost savings and health benefits, but the other incentives, too.

This was one of the hardest parts of Jeff's job. Some people wanted to be helped, but occasionally there was one who wasn't ready. It was generally a personal preference. The ones that did want to be helped seemed to love their jobs more, and got engaged with the process. They earned benefits, saved money, and added years to their lives.

"That's one of the most common myths I hear that prevent people from engaging in health and fitness," Jeff said. "That there aren't enough hours in the day. I know it's hard, but we all have the same amount of time."

Don thought about what the coach said. He had to admit that it all made sense. He was starting to think it would be a good idea.

"Okay okay, you've convinced me," Don said. "I'm tired of being sick, and I'm tired of feeling sluggish. I need to get healthy. Tell me what I need to do."

"Let's log into the system and get enrolled," Jeff said. "I'll walk you through it."

Don listened as Jeff walked him step-by-step through the online enrollment. Don spent time with the assessment answering the questions, and even though some made him uncomfortable he completed it, answering 20 or so questions. As he went through them, he actually started thinking about ways he could improve things in his life. At the end of the assessment he saw that he had gotten points for the activity, toward lowering his insurance premium.

Since he was just in the hospital, he had current bloodwork and was able to submit those results to get credit for doing a screening. Next, he'd schedule an appointment to get the rest of his preventive care done, and make sure he had a plan to never be back in the ER.

"I'm never going backwards again," he said to himself. "Never."

For the next several weeks Don followed the plan and logged onto the portal. He read the emails that arrived from the health management program and talked to the health coach regularly, working the steps to participate. Week one, after the assessment was completed, the coach reviewed the next steps in the program. Week two, Don had signed up for a targeted program on reducing cholesterol and how to choose the right foods and develop better habits. All in all he was on the right track. He began preparing lunch at home to bring to work with him, and Vickie snuck fruits and vegetables into the lunch bag.

Sometimes he slipped up and ate a candy bar from the gas station, but the difference was that for the first time in his life, making bad health choices didn't feel right. He felt guilty when he ate junk food, instead of satisfied. He still smoked occasionally, but he hated it when he did. He had seen memos about a new smoking cessation program and wondered if it was worth trying. Anything that could help him live longer and kick the habit, would be worth it.

Inside he felt his perspective shifting. He sat at his desk day after day, and found himself actually reading the emails from the CEO about the corporate health program. Sometimes they offered simple reminders to get preventive checkups. Other times they offered special webinars, challenges, or tips for staying healthy.

Don finally took time to reflect on the comments his clients had made throughout the years about his eating habits and the American culture in general. One supplier, a Japanese executive, mentioned how the American culture was going downhill, and how people seemed more obese now than ever. Obese! His client actually used that word. It embarrassed him. There was a health care crisis in America, and almost every major news media or magazine was reporting about it. Not only that, even his clients had noticed. He realized he had a blind spot about the choices he was making, but now he was determined to turn it around.

When Don watched the news at night he saw lots of stories about how American companies were less competitive and less productive and taxes kept going up to pay for the cost of healthcare. That resonated with him. Where were the good old days? People used to talk about American innovation. Now all of the stories of hot new companies came from booming economies like China and India. One report said that for the first time, half of all Americans were considered obese.

He decided he wasn't going to be one of them.

ELEVEN

Two years had passed. Angela walked into her office and spent the first couple of hours reading, having a healthy breakfast of oatmeal and fruit at her desk, and checking email.

She had learned from the wellness coach to spend equal time nurturing her emotional, physical, and intellectual wellness, and she remained committed to the process. Her reading list had grown to include self improvement books, and she was getting more sleep.

Later that night Angela stood in the kitchen after the run with her daughter and drank an entire bottle of water. Two years ago it would've been a diet soda, but her wellness coach had sent her a study that linked obesity to diet drinks. She spent time researching it, and was astounded at the facts. People who drank diet drinks had a much higher incidence of obesity as a group overall. And the information about the nations food supply was just as staggering. Angela spent time reading about the science of how food was grown, processed, and transported, learning about the chemicals that food companies added to create an addictive product. Things like sugar and salt were things that caused cravings, not unlike tobacco or alcohol. Angela had learned so much, and now she was making better choices.

A nutritionist from the program had even opened her eyes about buying organic vegetables and fruits that had to conform to higher standards. She learned that all foods were definitely not created equal. Some were actually harmful instead of nutritious!

Angela watched her daughter sit down at the kitchen table and open the laptop.

"Doing homework?" Angela asked.

"Nope. I'm going to write a letter to your boss."

"For what?"

Angela walked over, and looked over Jessica's shoulder. Sure enough she had her company web page up.

"I'm searching for his email address," Jessica said.

Angela laughed, "What on earth for?"

"Because I've got to thank him for giving me my mom back," she said. "You were working too much and I barely saw you. Now we jog every day!"

Angela laughed. Her daughter was right. Not only that, but those tests might just have saved her life. Her cholesterol had been high, and because of the preventive tests she had the knowledge to change it. She started eating less cheese, pasta, and red meat, and began incorporating vegetables into her life.

She believed more than ever, in the power of prevention.

She was determined to finish strong.

"I think he'd like that," she said.

The CEO had been committed to transforming his culture. Angela envisioned him opening a letter from a child. It would confirm he'd been right all along.

Not only did the program save lives and cut costs, but it changed families too. She owed a lot to the company for the health management program. In a lot of ways it was a wake up call, and it caused her to reevaluate their life. Everything they'd done in the past was putting their family on a trajectory of disease and obesity. She hadn't realized it but the long nights, fast food, and sedentary days were leading them both down a bad path. Now, Jessica was different. She was happier, more engaged at school, and had an interest in being active. She read health blogs on the Internet and even recruited her friends for runs! Angela was proud of how far they'd come. It had bonded them together as a family.

Across town, Don sat down to a meal with his wife and for the first time in a long time made healthy choices. He reached for the asparagus and added it to his plate, chuckling inside. Why had he stubbornly resisted for so long? Ultimately he had only been hurting himself.

Now he was completely mindful of every decision. A year ago he would've shunned anything green. But now he actually discovered that he liked broccoli, especially with a little bit of lemon on it, and he loved colorful peppers and salads. Things he'd never chosen before seemed appealing to him, mainly because he had become educated about new foods that made him feel more energetic, youthful, and vibrant. The incentives had driven him to make better choices through the health management program at work, because he'd wanted to reduce his insurance costs. But then he found that he actually liked the way he felt when he made those choices. And he wanted his family to be healthier too.

His entire mindset had changed, and it was hard to believe he'd come this far. In the end, it was the health coach who made him realize that he wasn't proving anything to anyone by being resistant to change. He was only hurting himself. When he started saving money on his health insurance premiums he was even more convinced.

This new path of living in health, getting regular checkups, and making better food choices would lead to a better life. Not just for him but for everyone.

The following day Don met the CEO for their regularly scheduled run in the parking lot of the office building. They had developed a routine of jogging a half mile on the wooded trail around campus, then running, then jogging again. By the third week John started bringing small five pound weights for them to carry, and the resistance helped him build muscle. At first it had been difficult, and Don could barely keep up. But now he was in as good a shape as his boss. His arms had toned up a lot, and he could start seeing muscle in his midsection again. In a lot of ways Don felt much leaner and healthier than he had twenty years before. Partnering with John had been good for him. They challenged each other, and week after week he enjoyed it more. He was beginning to see himself as an athlete, and not as that overweight pasty guy who binged on processed foods.

For John, it was nice to take the time to spend time with a friend again, instead of just golfing with clients or spending time in meetings pursuing business. There was no pressure to perform in front of Don. They were colleagues, and working towards the same goal.

"Can you actually believe it took us so long to do this?" John said. Their runs reminded him of the early days when he and Don had both led simpler lives. Now they had gotten back to the basics, and were focused on taking care of themselves first.

"I think I've finally discovered that there are no shortcuts to getting healthy" John said with a chuckle. "It's been drilled into me these last few months from our health care management program and of course I knew it all along, but in my own life I've realized that I just have to make the time to be healthy and make better choices."

"Agreed," Don said. "Why did it take us so long to realize it?"

"I think sometimes we get so caught up in getting more, achieving more, and obtaining that next level that we don't spend enough time in the moment. Just enjoying the moment we're in now."

Don stretched. He leaned forward, and felt his hamstring tighten. "You're right," he said, agreeing with his friend. "Most humans don't appreciate the life they have because they want the life they don't have. Most people grow up wanting. They want more. Because they grew up in a world where there's a lot available. I'm guilty of it. I always wanted more. More money, more power, more recognition. But in all that chasing I almost lost my life."

Don had lost thirty pounds so far. Now he could run a mile, which had been unthinkable a couple years ago. He shook his head. "It's crazy, isn't it?"

John smiled. "What's that?"

"To think that we humans need such a big wake up call to jolt us out of our patterns of chasing the wrong things, in order to recalibrate our focus back onto the right things."

"It seems crazy that we could neglect our health until it is in crisis mode, for sure," John said. "I'm just as guilty. I just didn't have a heart attack. Yet."

"There's a lot to be said for contentment, John. I mean, we can strive and achieve and build the biggest company, but in the end at some point we've got to stop, look around, and be grateful for what we've got."

"I'm finally content," John said. "It took me a long time but now that we've implemented a health management program I feel like we've created more than just a corporation. We've created a legacy. Something that will influence people to get healthy, and change generations."

Later that afternoon the CEO looked out his office window at the grounds surrounding his office building. The culture had transformed, and the way they worked and lived had changed too. He'd built a running course in the woods surrounding their building, and he'd changed the cafeteria choices to include healthy foods. His employees were participating in the health management program and their performance was strong. Some of their customers had even decided to do the same thing, and he had seen entire cultures of corporations now focusing on incorporating healthier lifestyle programs, preventive testing, and incentive programs to get their employees healthier. Participation in the first year had been 63%. By year two they were at 81% and just like the consultants had said, their health care costs had been reduced.

All of it had exceeded his expectations.

TWELVE

It had been been two years since they started the health management program.

Everything felt right, the culture had changed, and people were engaged.

There was a euphoria in the hallways, and as John walked through them on his way to the boardroom for the annual meeting he felt enthusiastic, not hesitant like he had in prior years.

They had made some good decisions for the company. John remembered back to the day they had made the decision to be proactive, stop being complacent, and get the workforce active and moving. It was like breathing new life into the culture. The smell, the feel, and the energy was all different. But would it translate into sustainably reduced cost?

John's team gathered in the fishbowl and took their familiar places at the conference table. An assistant distributed the report to every attendee. Like most reports and handouts, John wanted to have patience and let them present, but he couldn't help but flip to the last few pages. Were costs improving?

He got to the page on cost containment and saw a graph that showed that costs were now below the national averages. The program had reduced their expenses!

With a slight grin, he flipped back to page one and let the team present the findings report.

Surprisingly, Judy from HR stood first and gave a positive review of the program. When she was done, she turned to face him.

"I must admit I was skeptical about the change this

type of program would bring," she said. "But John, I must applaud your leadership and persistence in making this happen. Not only has employee participation been strong, but the program has been well received by our employees and it's actually made my job a lot easier. Turnover has been reduced!"

John smiled. Judy had been the hardest one to convince about the value of the program.

The CFO stood next. "This program has reduced the bottom line as well," he said, referring to the report. The team flipped the pages. "Look on page four," he said, "In year one costs rose slightly because so many employees adopted the program and took action to get their preventive tests. But as you can see, by the end of year two we started to see a downward slope. Compliance is up, and costs have gone down. They didn't rise at all this year and that's a first."

"What's the prediction for year three?" John asked.

"It's all positive. This was the first year we didn't have to budget for a 17% increase."

The consultant chimed in. "Judy, can you share the feedback from HR about hiring, and how the implementation of this program has impacted your department?"

Judy beamed. "Yes, the results have been great! We

are now viewed as a more attractive, competitive company to work for. Hiring is easier, and there are a lot more employee referrals now because we are viewed as a great place to work."

"How's absenteeism?" Asked the CFO.

"It was a problem in the past, quite frankly," Judy replied. "But now it's a half day less on average for an employee!"

John sat back in the chair and drew out a deep breath. For the first time in years he felt like they were on the right track. Presenter after presenter stood to give their respective departmental reports. All of it had exceeded their expectations. The program implementation had been a success. When the meeting adjourned, each team member shook his hand and congratulated him on a job well done. John walked back to his office, lowered himself into his comfortable chair, and stared out the window. He took a moment to feel grateful for everything he had and the employees who had helped him create success.

He turned, and opened his email.

He sorted through several until he came to one from a name he didn't recognize. The email was simple.

From: Jessica Davis

Thank you for giving me my mom back. We spend more time together now, because of your health program. It has changed my life.

Jessica, age 12
Daughter of Angela Davis

John felt a lump in his throat.

Now, reading the letter from a little girl whose life had been changed, his eyes welled. If one life was transformed, it had all been worth it. If a family had been changed, it was the culmination of a dream, and if a culture, or thousands of lives could be transformed into thinking and living and acting healthier, he knew that he'd been in that role for a purpose. All of the work he'd done was for a reason. Families could get healthier. Children would have more time with their parents. Companies would have less downtime, and reduced healthcare costs, and employees would live more balanced lives with less disease and more life.

He had known that the program would be beneficial for the company, but he never really realized how important it would be for the employees. It was a big decision, but now he was so glad he'd taken the leap and implemented it. John printed the email, and placed it on his desk as a reminder.

At the end of the day, it had all been worth it.

ABOUT THE AUTHOR

Michael Nadeau
Chief Executive Officer of Viverae, Inc.

Health care advocate Michael Nadeau is passionate about transforming health care in the United States. He founded Viverae, a performance-based health management company, as a solution to corporate Americas excessive utilization of health care plans and a generally unhealthy U.S. workforce.

A New England native, Nadeau began his career in the Northeast working in the software development, IT consulting and health care industries.

Nadeau has been recognized for his entrepreneurial spirit as a winner of the Ernst & Young Entrepreneur Of The Year® award. Under his leadership, Viverae has been recognized by *Inc.* magazine as one of the nations fastest growing companies, one of the Best Places to Work and one of the Healthiest Employers in Dallas, along with several other national and regional awards.

Nadeau is an expert in corporate health care solutions, health management programs, health risk identification and employee health incentives.

Good Health 24/7 starts from 9 to 5